27.99

D0321489

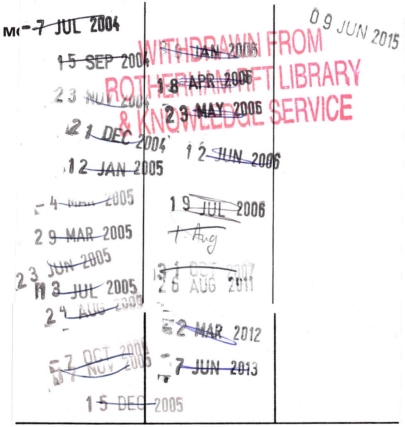
This book should be returned by the last date stamped above. You may renew the loan personally, by post or telephone for a further period if the book is not required by another reader.

QBASE ANAESTHESIA 6
MCQ COMPANION TO FUNDAMENTALS OF ANAESTHESIA

Colin Pinnock MBBS, FRCA
Consultant Anaesthetist
Alexandra Hospital
Redditch, Worcestershire

Robert Jones MRCA
Staff Grade Anaesthetist
Withybush Hospital, Haverfordwest

Simon Maguire MBChB, FRCA
Consultant Anaesthetist
South Manchester University Hospitals Trust
Wythenshawe, Manchester

Julian M. Barker MBChB, MRCP, FRCA
Consultant in Cardiothoracic Anaesthesia and Intensive Care
South Manchester University Hospitals Trust
Wythenshawe, Manchester

Simon Mills MBChB, MRCP, FRCA
Consultant Anaesthetist
Blackpool Victoria Hospital, Blackpool

QBase developed and edited by
Edward Hammond MA, BM, BCh, MRCP, FRCA
Consultant Anaesthetist
Royal Devon and Exeter Hospital, Exeter

GMM
London ♦ San Francisco

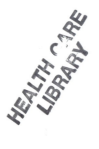

Greenwich Medical Media Limited
137 Euston Road, London
NW1 2AA

ISBN 1 84110 098 6

First Published 2004

Typeset by Mizpah Publishing Services, Chennai, India
Printed by Cromwell Press Ltd, Trowbridge

Contents

Preface

This book has been designed for use alongside the textbook 'Fundamentals of Anaesthesia' as a revision tool for candidates preparing for the Primary FRCA. The three topics of the primary MCQ paper are covered within and some extra clinical material has been included for those readers wishing to prepare themselves for the OSCE and Viva 2 parts of the examination. Questions have been carefully written to represent the sort of topics that may be met in the examination hall and the answers are accompanied by a reference to further reading where more detail may be obtained.

I am very grateful for the effort put in by my co-authors in the preparation of this manuscript. Collectively, we wish all candidates using this volume good luck in the examination and hope this modest work will help them on their way.

Colin Pinnock
Redditch
January 2004

QBase Anaesthesia on CD-ROM

MINIMUM SYSTEM REQUIREMENTS

- An IBM compatible PC with a 80386 processor and 4 MB of RAM
- VGA monitor set up to display at least 256 colours
- CD-ROM drive
- Windows 95 or higher with Microsoft compatible mouse

NB: The display setting of your computer must be set to display 'SMALL FONTS' (see MS Windows manuals for further instructions on how to do this if necessary)

INSTALLATION INSTRUCTIONS

The program will install the appropriate files onto your hard drive. It requires the QBase CD-ROM to be in installed in the CD-ROM drive (usually drives D: or E:)

In order to run QBase, the CD must be in the drive

Print **Readme.txt** and **Helpfile.txt** on the CD-ROM for fuller instructions and user manual

WINDOWS 95, 98, 2000, XP

1. Insert the QBase CD-ROM into the drive
2. From the Start Menu, select the Run... option, type **D:\setup.exe** (where D: is the CD-ROM drive) and press OK or **OR** open the contents of the CD-ROM and double-click the **setup.exe** icon
3. Follow the 'Full – install all files' to accept the default directory for installation of QBase
4. Click 'Yes' to the prompt 'Do you want setup to create Program Manager groups?' If you have a previously installed version of QBase, click 'Yes' to the next prompt 'Should the new Program Manager groups replace existing duplicate groups?'
5. To run QBase, go to the Start Menu, then Programs, QBase and **QBase Exam**. From Windows Explorer, double-click the **QBase.exe** file in the QBase folder on your hard drive.

Editor's Note

QBase Anaesthesia 6 has been designed as an MCQ Companion to the second edition of GMM's bestselling *Fundamentals of Anaesthesia*. If you have loaded previous versions of the QBase Anaesthesia series and are familiar with the program, you can start using it immediately. This CD contains the latest version of the QBase software and we suggest you install the program to update previous. Follow the installation instructions contained in the **Readme.txt** on the CD.

The book and CD contain 500 MCQ questions to test your knowledge prior to taking the Primary FRCA examination. There are 150 questions in Pharmacology, Physiology and Physics/Clinical Measurement as used in the exam. The Exam 1 to 5 buttons have been set up to provide a 90 question paper in the current format of the Primary FRCA MCQ examination. The Autoset exam option also chooses 90 questions, with 30 from each of the 3 core subjects used in the actual exam. You can, of course, choose any combination of subjects and number of questions to set up your own exam for revision or assessment. The CD also contains 50 Clinical questions following the format of *Fundamentals of Anaesthesia*. These are not selected in the Autoset exam option, but are there to test your ability to apply your knowledge of the core subjects to 'real' clinical situations.

This latest set of MCQ questions, in conjunction with the QBase Program and *Fundamentals of Anaesthesia*, will help you prepare for the Primary FRCA. QBase will assist you in assessing your exam technique and the effect of this on your overall performance in the MCQ.

The Royal College of Anaesthetists (RCA) has always advised candidates taking negatively MCQ exams not to guess, as this will result in a loss of marks. More recently, the RCA seems to have accepted that this may not be the case and that most candidates will benefit by at least including their 'educated guesses'. Our experience in teaching MCQ technique for the last 10 years shows that most candidates benefit from even 'wild guesses'. Some may lose a few marks. QBase is a tool designed to help you determine whether you are one of those that may lose marks and therefore should avoid guessing. Use it wisely – it is about what you do and *not* what other people do!

Good luck!

Edward Hammond
January 2004

List of Abbreviations

ACE   Angiotensin converting enzyme
ACTH   Adrenocorticotropic hormone
ADH   Anti-diuretic hormone
ADP   Adenosine diphosphate
AER   Auditory evoke responses
AIP   Acute intermittent porphyria
ALA   Aminolevulinic acid
ANP   Atrial natriuretic peptide
ANS   Autonomic nervous system
APTT   Activated partial thromboplastin time
ATP   Adenosine triphosphate

BMR   Basal metabolic rate

CBF   Cerebral blood flow
CNS   Central nervous system
COHb   Carboxyhaemoglobin
COPD   Chronic obstructive pulmonary disease
CPR   Cardiac pulmonary resuscitation
CRH   Corticotropin releasing hormone
CRO   Cathode ray oscilloscope
CSF   Cerebrospinal fluid
CTZ   Chemoreceptor trigger zone
CVP   Central venous pressure

DIC   Disseminated intravascular coagulation
DOPA   Dihydroxyphenylalanine
DVT   Deep venous thrombosis

ECF   Extracellular fluid
EEG   Electroencephalogram
EMA   Electromyogram
$ETCO_2$ End-tidal carbon dioxide

Fab   Antibody fragments
FEV   Forced expiratory volume
FFA   Free fatty acids
FFP   Fresh frozen plasma
FRC   Functional residual capacity
FSH   Follicle stimulating hormone

GABA   Gamma-aminobutyric acid
GFR   Glomerular filtration rate
GH   Growth hormone
GnRH   Gonadotrophin releasing hormone

HAFOE	High air flow oxygen enriched
HELLP	Hemolysis, elevated liver enzymes and low platelets
ICF	Intracellular fluid
IOP	Intraocular pressure
IPPV	Intermittent positive pressure ventilation
IVC	Inferior vena cava
IVRA	Intravenous regional anaesthesia
Laser	Light amplification by simulated emission of radiation
LCD	Liquid crystal display
LED	Light emitting diode
LH	Luteinising hormone
LVEDP	Left ventricular end diastolic pressure
MAC	Minimum alveolar concentration
MAO	Monoamine oxidase
MAOI	Monoamine oxidase inhibitor
MAP	Mean arterial pressure
MH	Malignant hyperthermia
MI	Myocardial infarction
NMDA	N-methyl, D-aspartate
NSAID	Non-steroidal anti-inflammatory drug
PAH	Para-aminohippuric acid
PEEP	Positive end expiratory pressure
PEFR	Peak expiratory flow rate
PNMT	Phenylethanolamine-N-methyltransferase
pO_2	Partial pressure of oxygen
PT	Prothrombin time
PVR	Pulmonary vascular resistance
RPF	Renal plasma flow
SCD	Sickle cell disease
SLE	Systemic lupus erythematosus
SVP	Saturated vapour pressure
SVR	Systemic vascular resistance
TBW	Total body water
TNF	Tumour necrosis factor
TOF	Train-of-four
TSH	Thyroid stimulating hormone
VER	Visual evoke responses
VIE	Vacuum-insulated evaporator

Section 1 – Questions

Physics and Clinical Measurement

Questions

Q 1. With respect to damping

A. Damping does not apply to electrical devices
B. Damping affects the step response of the system
C. Underdamping results in overestimation
D. Overdamping results in overestimation
E. Critical damping refers to the fastest steady state reading of the system with no oscillation

Q 2. Concerning the gas laws

A. Boyle's law refers to the relationship between temperature and pressure of a gas
B. Temperature is measured on the absolute temperature scale
C. Temperature is a constant in Charles' law
D. Boyle's law states that at a constant volume, pressure varies with temperature
E. The gas laws are only true for air

Q 3. The critical temperature of a gas is that

A. Below which it solidifies
B. Above which it will not liquefy despite increased pressure
C. At which it sublimes
D. At which it liquefies if pressure is decreased
E. At which kinetic energy is zero

Q 4. The following are correct SI Units

A. The unit of energy is newton
B. The unit of power is watt
C. The unit of frequency is hertz
D. The unit of mass is gram
E. The unit of length is metre

Q 5. **The peak expiratory flow rate (PEFR)**

A. In normal adults is often more than 500 l/min
B. Can be measured by a pneumotachograph
C. Can be measured by the Wright's peak flow meter
D. Increases with age
E. Can be improved by training

Q 6. **The amount of gas dissolved in a liquid**

A. Increases as the temperature of the liquid increases
B. Is proportional to the pressure of the gas in contact with the liquid
C. Is influenced by the presence of other dissolved gases
D. Exerts the same 'tension' as the partial pressure of the gas in contact with the liquid at equilibrium
E. Is proportional to the molecular weight of the gas

Q 7. **The laminar flow of a gas through a tube is**

A. Proportional to the square root of the pressure drop along the tube
B. Proportional to the length of the tube
C. Proportional to the fourth power of the diameter
D. Inversely proportional to the square of the viscosity of the gas
E. Inversely proportional to the square root of the density of the gas

Q 8. **A thermistor**

A. Is a type of transducer
B. Comprises a junction of dissimilar metals
C. Is used for electrical measurement of temperature
D. Can be used in a Wheatstone bridge circuit
E. Is very delicate

Q 9. **The following are derived SI units**

A. pascal
B. hertz
C. joule

D. newton

E. coulomb

Q 10. When five 2 V batteries are joined in series across a resistance of 1 megaohm the current flowing in the circuit is

A. 0.2 A

B. 0.01 mA

C. 0.001 A

D. 0.00001 A

E. 0.005 mA

Q 11. Critical temperature is

A. The temperature at which a liquid will change into a vapour without heat being required

B. The temperature above which a gas cannot be liquefied by pressure

C. The temperature at which latent heat of vapourisation becomes maximal

D. The temperature at which latent heat of vapourisation becomes zero

E. The temperature above which a substance cannot exist in a liquid state

Q 12. Vapour concentration in a breathing system may be monitored by

A. Infrared gas analysis

B. Ultraviolet gas analysis

C. Paramagnetism

D. Mass spectrometry

E. Gas chromatography

Q 13. Pressure gauges on anaesthetic machines

A. Are calibrated in newtons

B. Control flow rate

C. Can be used to measure gas flow

D. Work on the principle of the Bourdon gauge

E. Reduce high to low pressure

Q 14. The following affect turbulent flow

    A. Length of tube
    B. Radius of tube
    C. Drop in pressure
    D. Density of fluid
    E. Viscosity of fluid

Q 15. Latent heat of vapourisation

    A. Is lower at high temperatures
    B. Is the energy required to change a liquid to a vapour without a change in temperature
    C. Is zero at the critical temperature
    D. SI units are joule/kg
    E. Is responsible for the majority of heat loss from the respiratory tract

Q 16. Surgical diathermy

    A. Requires a large plate area
    B. Uses a sinusoidal waveform
    C. Requires the plate to be sited over an area with good blood supply
    D. Operates at frequencies below 400 kHz
    E. Always requires an earth

Q 17. With respect to humidifiers

    A. Ideal droplet size is one micron diameter
    B. There may be a risk of scalding
    C. The Bernoulli effect may be employed
    D. Water baths are more efficient than nebulisers
    E. Infection may be introduced

Q 18. Boyle's law relates to

    A. Ideal gases only
    B. Pressure and volume
    C. Constant temperature
    D. Boyle's bottle
    E. An inverse relationship between pressure and volume

Q 19. Cooling during surgery can be decreased by

    A. Ambient theatre temperature of 20°C
    B. Space blankets
    C. Warmed intravenous fluids
    D. Phenothiazines
    E. Humidified gases

Q 20. One mole of a gas

    A. Occupies 22.4 l at room temperature
    B. Has the same volume for any gas
    C. Contains Avogadro's number of molecules
    D. May be liquefied by compression if above critical temperature
    E. Is one gram molecular weight

Q 21. A rise in temperature

    A. Increases liquid vapourisation
    B. Can be measured by a Bourdon gauge
    C. Increases the amount of gas dissolved in a liquid
    D. Moves the oxyhaemoglobin saturation curve to the left
    E. Is related to saturated vapour pressure (SVP)

Q 22. The rate of gas diffusion through a membrane is directly proportional to

    A. Pressure
    B. Membrane surface area
    C. Membrane thickness
    D. Gas molecular weight
    E. Gas solubility

Q 23. A thermistor

    A. Demonstrates the Seebeck effect
    B. Shows a linear relationship between resistance and temperature
    C. Has a resistance that changes with time
    D. Exhibits hysteresis
    E. Has a negative temperature coefficient of resistance

Q 24. Pressure

A. Relates force to area
B. Relates flow to area
C. Can be measured by a column of fluid
D. SI unit is newtons per square metre
E. Is the force acting per unit mass

Q 25. The following are fundamental SI units

A. Degree Celsius
B. Candela
C. Metre per second
D. Ampere
E. Mole

Q 26. Concerning pulse oximetry

A. Oxyhaemoglobin and deoxyhaemoglobin light absorption is equal at the isobestic point of 660 nm
B. Measurements are accurate in the presence of carboxyhaemoglobin
C. Measurements are accurate in the presence of high levels of bilirubin
D. Measurements are accurate in the presence of pigmented skin
E. Saturation of venous blood may be recorded

Q 27. Surgical diathermy

A. Commonly delivers 1 kW of power
B. Operates at frequencies around 10 kHz
C. Requires good contact of the indifferent electrode
D. May be unipolar or bipolar
E. May be safely used on patients having cardiac pacemakers

Q 28. With respect to electrical equipment

A. Double insulated equipment can be used in wet areas
B. Class 1 equipment is double insulated
C. The patient should be connected to earth
D. Class 2 equipment is fully earthed
E. Class 3 equipment is low voltage

Q 29. With respect to humidity

   A. Absolute humidity is independent of temperature
   B. Relative humidity is independent of temperature
   C. Relative humidity in the operating theatre should exceed 50%
   D. Humidity may be measured by electrical transducers
   E. Regnault's hygrometer uses a hair

Q 30. Doppler ultrasound

   A. Uses transducer crystals to transmit and receive ultrasound
   B. Transducers may be placed directly on the skin
   C. Can be used to measure blood pressure
   D. Is unaffected by movement
   E. Measurements are affected by diathermy

Q 31. When gas flows through a tube

   A. Laminar flow implies that flow is smooth and parallel to the wave of the tube
   B. With laminar flow, resistance is inversely proportional to the diameter of the tube
   C. Above the critical flow rate, turbulent flow results
   D. At a restriction, sharp curve or valve, turbulent flow develops
   E. When turbulent flow develops, flow is inversely proportional to the square of the gas density

Q 32. Regarding biological signals

   A. EEG signals have a voltage of 50 mV
   B. EEG signals have frequencies up to 60 Hz
   C. ECG signals have voltages of 0.1–500 mV
   D. EMG signals may extend up to 1 kHz
   E. Signal-to-noise ratio is the ratio of noise amplitude to signal amplitude expressed in decibels

Q 33. With respect to the measurement of gas flow

   A. The rotating bobbin is an example of a constant orifice device
   B. The Fleisch pneumotachograph is an example of a variable orifice flowmeter

C. Gases which have the same density will give similar readings in a rotating bobbin flowmeter at high flows
D. If a bobbin does not spin, the reading will be inaccurate
E. At the narrowest part of a Venturi, the pressure of gas will fall

Q 34. The following are true of an ideal gas

A. The volume of a given mass of gas at a given pressure is inversely proportional to its temperature
B. At constant temperature, the volume of a given mass of gas is directly proportional to its pressure
C. At absolute zero, the volume of a gas would be one volume percent
D. At a given temperature and pressure, one mole of any gas occupies the same volume as one mole of any other gas
E. The ideal Gas law is a combination of Boyle's and Charles' laws

Q 35. Humidity

A. Expressed in absolute units, relates the amount of water present to the maximum amount possible at that temperature
B. Expressed in absolute units, is the mass of water in unit volume of gas at standard temperature and pressure
C. Is a measure of the total water content in the gas, both vapour and droplets
D. Expressed in relative units, compares the humidity at ambient temperature to that at absolute zero
E. In the lungs is usually 95–100% of the maximum possible

Q 36. Sources of error in arterial pressure monitoring include

A. Air bubbles
B. Rigid catheters
C. Blood clots
D. Lack of a zero point
E. Transducers with a high frequency response

Q 37. The following are true of methods of oxygen analysis

A. A paramagnetic analyser measures the percentage of oxygen in the analysed gas

B. A mass spectrometer is rendered inaccurate by the presence of nitrous oxide

C. Infrared absorption can be used for breath-by-breath analysis

D. The Haldane method is inaccurate in the presence of nitrous oxide

E. The polarographic method consumes oxygen

Q 38. The following properties may be used to measure the concentration of a gas or vapour

A. The refractive index

B. The thermal conductivity

C. The solubility

D. Light emission

E. Light absorption

Q 39. Lasers

A. Are high power devices

B. Contain diffuse light waves

C. Contain light waves that are in phase

D. Are classified 1–4, 4 being least dangerous

E. May cause a fire hazard

Q 40. The following physical properties may be used in the measurement of pressure

A. Change of electrical resistance in a wire

B. Variable inductance

C. Focusing of light

D. Change in flow through a narrow tube

E. Torricellian vacuum

Q 41. The Wheatstone bridge circuit

A. Can be used to measure changes in resistance

B. Is insensitive to small changes in resistance

C. Cannot measure capacitance

D. Gives a non-linear output
E. Depends upon the ratio of the two resistances in one limb of the circuit compared to the ratio of the two resistances in the other limb

Q 42. Ohm's law

A. Can only be applied to direct current circuits
B. Can be used to derive the power of a circuit
C. Suggests that resistances in parallel are additive
D. Suggests that the current through a light bulb is proportional to the voltage
E. Suggests that the potential differences across each of two resistors in a series circuit will be in the same proportion as their resistance

Q 43. The following are basic SI units

A. Metre
B. Kelvin
C. Pascal
D. Watt
E. Coulomb

Q 44. Pressure

A. Is defined as force per unit area
B. Has the same units as work
C. Has the same units as rate of work
D. The SI unit is the pascal
E. May be measured with a manometer

Q 45. The following statements are true about laminar flow

A. The fluid has a conical front end
B. It depends on viscosity of the fluid
C. It depends on density of the fluid
D. It depends on the tube being straight
E. Laminar flow occurs in the trachea during quiet breathing

Q 46. An inductor

- **A.** Can be constructed of wire wound around an aluminium core
- **B.** Has no effect on a steady current
- **C.** Impedance increases with increasing frequency of alternating current
- **D.** Maximum current occurs as an alternating voltage passes through zero
- **E.** Has a high resistance to steady current

Q 47. Laminar flow through a cannula is directly proportional to

- **A.** Temperature
- **B.** Viscosity of the fluid
- **C.** Ambient pressure
- **D.** Length of the cannula
- **E.** The square of the radius of the cannula

Q 48. Factors which affect the resistance to flow of a fluid include

- **A.** Viscosity
- **B.** Density
- **C.** Temperature
- **D.** Osmolality
- **E.** Surface tension

Q 49. The surface tension of a liquid

- **A.** Is related to the temperature of the liquid
- **B.** Is related to the viscosity of the liquid
- **C.** Is related to the radius of the droplet
- **D.** Is measured in kPa/m
- **E.** Is a pressure

Q 50. The cathode ray oscilloscope

- **A.** Horizontal deflection represents the timebase
- **B.** Timebase is created using a constant voltage electrode
- **C.** Does not emit radiation
- **D.** Does not create an electrostatic charge
- **E.** Does not differentiate between alternating current and direct current

Q 51. Blood viscosity depends on

- **A.** Temperature
- **B.** Plasma proteins
- **C.** Age
- **D.** Haemoglobin concentration
- **E.** Systolic blood pressure

Q 52. Viscosity

- **A.** Can be measured by a dual drum technique
- **B.** Is temperature-dependent
- **C.** Is dependent on intermolecular attraction
- **D.** The unit is the poise
- **E.** Can be measured using a viscometer

Q 53. Regarding sound waves

- **A.** The decibel is a unit on a linear scale
- **B.** The decibel is the SI unit of sound measurement
- **C.** Sound is painful to humans over 75 decibels
- **D.** The human auditory range is 20–25,000 Hz
- **E.** Sound waves can be focused using acoustic lenses

Q 54. The venturi effect

- **A.** Is used in ventilator design
- **B.** Is used to enrich atmospheric air
- **C.** Depends upon the pressure-lowering effect of gas flowing through a narrowed tube
- **D.** Is applicable only to gases
- **E.** May be used to test breathing systems

Q 55. The Coanda effect is

- **A.** A venturi effect
- **B.** Employed in fluidic switching in ventilator design
- **C.** Caused by an increase in flow and a drop in pressure when gas is passed through a constrictor
- **D.** Caused by an increase in flow and an increase in pressure when gas is passed through a constrictor
- **E.** Seen in constricted blood vessels

Q 56. In a variable performance face mask

A. High patient inspiratory flow rate reduces oxygen concentration
B. Oxygen concentration increases during an expiratory pause
C. Carbon dioxide concentration increases during an expiratory pause
D. Side holes allow venting of expired gases and entrainment of air
E. Inspired concentration of oxygen is independent of oxygen flow rate

Q 57. With a fixed performance mask such as a Ventimask

A. Rebreathing is possible
B. Plugging the side-holes increases the oxygen concentration
C. Increase in oxygen concentration requires higher oxygen flows
D. There is a high equipment dead space
E. The total gas flow is higher than the patient's peak expiratory flow

Q 58. Flow can be measured by

A. Pressure drop across an orifice
B. The Fick principle
C. High frequency sound wave reflection
D. Spinning vane
E. Bubble flowmeters

Q 59. The electromagnetic flowmeter

A. Depends on the Ohm's law of electromagnetic induction
B. Has two probes – one electric and one magnetic
C. Is more accurate using AC than DC
D. Can be incorporated in an intravascular probe
E. Can be used for transcutaneous measurement of blood flow in vessels

Q 60. Concerning variable orifice flowmeters

A. The tube must be slightly inclined to the vertical to avoid friction
B. There is a constant pressure drop across the bobbin

C. The bobbin is scored to avoid friction

D. Are accurate only for laminar flow

E. An orifice has a diameter shorter than its length

Q 61. Regarding indirect measurement of blood pressure

A. Automated oscillometry machines over read at high pressures

B. Infrared plethysmography can be utilised

C. The Doppler principle can be utilised

D. Oscillotonometry machines detect Korotkov sounds

E. Automated oscillometry machines inflate to 100 mmHg above systolic pressure

Q 62. With regard to capnography

A. End-tidal carbon dioxide concentration exceeds arterial

B. Most clinical instruments are based on infrared spectrophotometry

C. Sidestream capnographs sample at 600 ml/min

D. In sidestream capnographs the head is the sampling chamber

E. Mainstream capnographs have a slow response time

Q 63. The pneumotachograph

A. Is affected by temperature

B. Gives direct reading of pressure drop

C. Must have a small resistance to keep the flow laminar

D. Permits breath-by-breath analysis

E. Is affected by viscosity

Q 64. The following are appropriate methods of measurement

A. Total body water by using deuterium oxide

B. RBC mass by radioactivity

C. ECF by radio-labelled albumin

D. ICF = ECF − TBW

E. Plasma volume by radio-labelled albumin

Q 65. Measurement of the extracellular fluid compartment may be achieved by using

  A. Radio-labelled albumin
  B. Sucrose
  C. Radio-labelled sulphate
  D. Deuterium oxide
  E. Inulin

Q 66. The following are analogue methods of signal display

  A. Light emitting diodes (LED)
  B. Liquid crystal display (LCD)
  C. Oscilloscope
  D. Chart recorder
  E. Galvanometer

Q 67. The following accurately measure respiratory volumes

  A. Wright's peak flow meter
  B. Wet spirometer
  C. Benedict-Roth spirometer
  D. Vitalograph
  E. Pneumotachograph

Q 68. The following measure volume by flow-volume loops

  A. Wright's respirometer
  B. Peak flow meter
  C. Pneumotachograph
  D. Vitalograph
  E. Benedict-Roth spirometer

Q 69. A Wright's respirometer over-reads

  A. If placed on a catheter mount
  B. If low gas flows are used
  C. If nitrogen dioxide is used
  D. If higher than 30% oxygen is used
  E. If the vanes are wet

Q 70. Concerning humidification of gases

A. The absolute humidity of air at 37°C is 44 mg/l

B. HMEs achieve relative humidity of 85%

C. Hot water bath humidifiers are prone to bacterial colonisation

D. In nebulised humidifiers droplets of 4 microns in size fall back into the container

E. Droplets of 1 micron or less may be produced by an ultrasonic nebuliser

Q 71. Boyle's law

A. Refers to a given mass of gas

B. States that pressure is inversely proportional to volume at constant temperature

C. Assumes an ideal gas

D. Compares changes in pressure with changes in temperature

E. Requires a constant volume of gas

Q 72. One gram molecular weight of a gas

A. Occupies a constant volume at room temperature

B. Is one mole

C. Contains a specific number of molecules whatever the temperature

D. Occupies 22.4 l at standard temperature and pressure

E. Contains Avogadro's number of molecules

Q 73. Critical temperature

A. Is the temperature above which a liquid boils

B. Is the temperature above which a liquid cannot be compressed

C. Is the temperature at which there is the least attraction between molecules

D. For oxygen is 36.5°C

E. Is identical to critical pressure

Q 74. Critical Pressure

A. Is the pressure above which a gas cannot be liquefied however much pressure is applied
B. Of oxygen is 20 bar
C. Is the pressure of a gas at its critical temperature
D. For nitrous oxide is 72 bar
E. Is the pressure required to liquefy a vapour at its critical temperature

Q 75. Concerning the use of the cryoprobe

A. It uses an adiabatic process
B. The sudden expansion of gas causes cooling to occur
C. Carbon dioxide is commonly used
D. It needs a temperature of $-90°C$ to be medically effective
E. Nitrogen dioxide may be used

Q 76. An exponential decay process

A. Decreases by constant proportion
B. Is 37% complete in one time constant
C. Half-life is half a time constant
D. Is 95% complete by three time constants
E. Has a constant half-life

Q 77. SVP depends on

A. Ambient temperature
B. Ambient pressure
C. Boiling point
D. The partial pressure of the gas above the liquid
E. Molecular weight of the liquid

Q 78. The vacuum-insulated evaporator (VIE)

A. Has a temperature inside of $-118°C$
B. Oxygen gas is supplied through the top of the VIE only
C. Has a safety valve that opens at approximately 1,700 kPa
D. Liquid oxygen is evaporated by passing it through copper superheaters in times of increased demand
E. The amount of oxygen remaining within the VIE is measured by a Bourdon pressure gauge

Q 79. Nitrous oxide

A. Has a critical temperature of 36.5°C
B. At temperatures above the critical temperature the plotted isotherm will follow Boyle's law
C. At temperatures below its critical temperature nitrous oxide exists as a liquid at high pressure
D. Does not support combustion
E. Is contained within size E cylinders on the back of anaesthetic machines

Q 80. The carbon dioxide electrode

A. Is unstable
B. Uses a lead anode
C. Relies on the carbonic acid equilibrium
D. Uses a silver/silver chloride reference electrode
E. Is also called a Clarke electrode

Q 81. Air contains

A. 78% nitrogen
B. 10% argon
C. 1% carbon dioxide
D. Water vapour
E. 5% xenon

Q 82. Latent heat

A. Is the energy required to change the state of a material
B. Requires a change in temperature
C. Is less at lower temperatures
D. Is greater at higher temperatures
E. Specific latent heat specifies a particular pressure

Q 83. Heat capacity

A. Is the energy required to cause a change of state
B. Is the same as latent heat
C. Is the energy required to raise the temperature of a body
D. Is Q/T where Q is the amount of heat energy and T is the temperature rise in degrees Celsius
E. Specific heat capacity is the amount of heat energy required to warm a body of 1 kg by 1°C

Q 84. Carbon dioxide diffuses through cell membranes more rapidly than oxygen because

A. It is more soluble
B. It has a different charge than oxygen
C. It has an active transport mechanism
D. It is a smaller molecule
E. There is a greater concentration gradient across the membrane

Q 85. With respect to diffusion of gases

A. Nitrous oxide and nitrogen have similar solubility
B. Diffusion is temperature dependent
C. Diffusion increases with membrane area
D. Diffusion varies with changes in pressure
E. Diffusion obeys Graham's law

Q 86. The rate of diffusion of a gas across a membrane depends on

A. The pressure gradient across the membrane
B. The density of the gas
C. The square of the molecular weight of the gas
D. Ambient temperature
E. Membrane thickness

Q 87. Regarding osmolality

A. It is measured by freezing point depression
B. It affects the SVP of the solvent
C. Plasma osmolality is mainly due to proteins
D. Normal plasma freezes at $-1°C$
E. Is defined as the number of osmoles per kilogram solvent

Q 88. Osmolality

A. Is measured in osmoles/l
B. Is related to the valency of the ions present
C. Of a body fluid is usually lower than its osmolarity
D. Is measured by the depression of freezing point
E. Is controlled by osmoreceptors in the hypothalamus

Q 89. Regarding temperature measurement

A. Mercury solidifies at −39°C
B. Alcohol boils at 55°C
C. One kelvin is 1/273.15°C
D. The triple point of water is 0.15°C
E. Absolute zero is −273.15°C

Q 90. Increases in temperature will cause

A. Increased viscosity of blood
B. Increased vaporisation of a volatile liquid
C. Increased resistance of a thermocouple
D. Increased solubility of carbon dioxide
E. Increase in output of a thermistor

Q 91. In ECG monitoring

A. Silver/silver chloride electrodes are used
B. Interference can be due to mains frequency
C. The CM5 configuration detects 90% of S-T segment changes due to left ventricular ischaemia
D. For CM5 the right arm electrode should be placed over the manubrium
E. The 'left arm' electrode should be placed over the apex of the heart

Q 92. Temperature loss from the body

A. Occurs due to convection of warm air next to the body
B. Sweating can increase heat loss by a factor of ten
C. Radiation losses can be decreased by the use of silver foil
D. Losses due to sweating decrease with increasing humidity
E. Occurs mainly through the hands and feet in children

Q 93. Hypothermia

A. Is defined by a core temperature of less than 34°C
B. Can result from exposure of tissue surfaces
C. Re-warming from 20°C must be passive
D. Shivering can increase metabolic rate by 600%
E. Bradycardia with hypertension will occur

Q 94. The thermistor in cardiac output measurement

A. Is distal to the PA catheter balloon
B. Becomes less accurate after 48 h in situ
C. Is not accurate to within 1°C
D. Measures core temperature
E. Is a semiconductor

Q 95. A thermistor

A. Reacts more quickly than a thermocouple
B. Can be used to measure blood flow
C. Exhibits the Seebeck effect
D. Has resistance which changes linearly with temperature
E. Has a high thermal capacity

Q 96. Specific latent heat

A. Is specified for 1 g of substance
B. Depends on ambient temperature
C. Depends on the mass of substance present
D. Is zero at critical temperature
E. Is lower at lower temperatures

Q 97. Wright's respirometer

A. Directly measures flow
B. Is an anemometer
C. Can record volumes up to 1,500 l
D. Is unaffected by humidity
E. Is unidirectional

Q 98. Humidity can be measured by

A. Biological tissue
B. The dew point
C. Electrical transducers
D. Mass spectrometry
E. Weighing

Q 99. Relative humidity

    A. Is the mass of water vapour present in a sample
    B. Can be measured with a hair hygrometer
    C. Is the same as absolute humidity
    D. Is constant within the nose
    E. Can be expressed as a ratio of vapour pressures

Q 100. Concerning electrical safety

    A. Diathermy machines always require earthing
    B. Wetness decrease resistance
    C. Induced current is reduced by using saline to prime manometer tubing
    D. A current below 24 mA is safe at the myocardium
    E. Risk of shock is increased with diathermy using floating patient circuits

Q 101. Concerning electrical safety

    A. The operating table should be earthed
    B. An intracardiac shock of 150 μA can cause asystolic cardiac arrest
    C. Earthed mains equipment will always have a leakage current to earth
    D. Ventricular fibrillation can be caused by a 50 mA current
    E. Wet hands decrease resistance

Q 102. The risk of AC electric shock is reduced by

    A. A conducting floor
    B. Conducting shoes
    C. A humid atmosphere
    D. Using bipolar diathermy
    E. Electrically isolated patient

Q 103. Regarding surgical diathermy

    A. High frequency current is necessary for its action
    B. The same frequency of current flows through the return plate as through the forceps
    C. If the return plate is detached from the patient no current will flow

D. There is a risk of burning the patient at the plate since the same current passes through the plate as through the patient

E. Earthing is still required even if bipolar forceps are used

Q 104. The following statements about biological potentials are true

A. ECG signals are in the range 1–2 mV
B. EMG signals are in the range 0.01–100 mV
C. EMG signals lie in the frequency range 100–1,000 Hz
D. ECG measures difference in potentials
E. EEG signals are in the range 6–9 μV

Q 105. The Kelvin scale

A. Measures energy
B. Has 273 degrees
C. Defines the boiling point of water as 373 degrees
D. Is the same as the Celsius scale
E. Defines the triple point of water as 273 degrees

Q 106. The following convert mechanical energy to electrical energy

A. Amplifiers
B. Transistors
C. Transducers
D. Photoelectric cells
E. Oscilloscope

Q 107. The following are types of transducers

A. Sphygmomanometer
B. Microphone
C. Strain gauge
D. Thermocouple
E. Oscilloscope

Q 108. A strain gauge can measure

A. Air flow
B. Light absorption

C. Blood flow

D. Air pressure

E. Mass

Q 109. Amplifiers

A. May contain transistors or valves

B. Change energy from one form to another

C. Increase amplitude of both noise and signals

D. May be non-linear

E. Are necessary to record most biological signals

Q 110. The cathode ray oscilloscope (CRO)

A. Is deflected in the x-axis by applying saw-tooth potential

B. When used to display the ECG is calibrated at 1 mm for 1 mV

C. Has a memory using digital storage

D. Displays information by splitting the incoming signal into fragments, storing them and then projecting them onto the screen

E. Is always monochromatic

Q 111. A nerve stimulator

A. Produces a current of 150 mA

B. Generates a square waveform

C. Electrodes implanted intradermally reduce impedance

D. Produces tetanic stimulation at 50 Hz

E. Uses 2 Hz stimulus for 200 ms to examine the TOF

Q 112. Accurate measurement of direct arterial blood pressure requires

A. Critical damping of 0.6

B. The use of a stiff diaphragm/transducer

C. The cannula to be compliant

D. The resonant frequency of the system should be greater than 40 Hz

E. Wide bore tubing

Q 113. Overdamping of a system will occur with

    A. An air bubble in the connecting tubing
    B. More than one 3-way tap in the connecting tubing
    C. Elastic tubing
    D. A non-functioning flushing system
    E. A silicone transducer

Q 114. A sphygmomanometer will overestimate blood pressure if

    A. The cuff is too wide
    B. The patient is obese
    C. Deflation of the cuff takes place too slowly
    D. The mercury manometer is placed above the level of the arm
    E. The patient has atrial fibrillation

Q 115. The Penaz technique

    A. Is invasive
    B. Uses plethysmography
    C. Does not require a pneumatic cuff
    D. Is suitable in the presence of peripheral vascular disease
    E. May be uncomfortable

Q 116. With regard to neuromuscular monitoring

    A. Train-of-four is 4 stimuli at 1 Hz
    B. Tetanic stimulation is used at 25 and 100 Hz
    C. Single twitch is delivered at 1 Hz
    D. Double burst consists of two tetanic periods of 50 Hz
    E. T4/T1 ratio should exceed 90% for adequate respiration

Q 117. The following may be used for monitoring of anaesthetic depth

    A. Evan's system
    B. Oesophageal contractility
    C. Evoked responses
    D. Spectral array
    E. Tunstall's technique

Q 118. Regarding pulse oximetry

 A. Anaemia causes under-reading
 B. Ambient light may cause interference
 C. It is inaccurate if arterial saturation reading is less than 70%
 D. Presence of carboxyhaemoglobin causes under-reading
 E. Two LEDs are needed

Q 119. Capnography

 A. Is the same as capnometry
 B. May utilise spectroscopy
 C. Is a discrete measurement
 D. Requires instruments with a short response time
 E. Shows a steep upward slope in COPD

Q 120. Paramagnetic analysers

 A. Measures all diamagnetic gases
 B. Use the principle of null deflection
 C. Have dumb-bell analysers which are filled with nitrogen
 D. Have a fast response time
 E. Are useful in measuring exhaled nitrogen

Q 121. The polarographic electrode

 A. Measures blood oxygen tension
 B. Has a platinum anode and silver/silver chloride cathode
 C. Has a voltage of 0.6 V applied between the electrodes
 D. Requires a constant temperature
 E. May be rendered inaccurate in the presence of halothane

Q 122. The Severinghaus electrode

 A. Is affected by nitrous oxide
 B. Is affected by temperature
 C. Contains glass which is permeable to carbon dioxide
 D. Contains sodium bicarbonate solution
 E. Contains glass permeable to hydrogen ions

Q 123. Rotameters

- **A.** Depend on laminar flow for their accuracy
- **B.** Will only function when upright
- **C.** Are constant pressure drop – constant orifice devices
- **D.** Are unaffected by static electricity
- **E.** Are not accurate below 1 l/min

Q 124. With respect to capnography

- **A.** Mainstream analysis is slower
- **B.** Sidestream analysis incurs dilution errors
- **C.** Sidestream analysers have dead space
- **D.** Sidestream analysers require water traps
- **E.** Infrared systems are the most frequently employed clinically

Q 125. Expired carbon dioxide as measured by a capnograph

- **A.** Increases with malignant hyperpyrexia
- **B.** Increases with pulmonary emboli
- **C.** Increases with exercise
- **D.** Can be used as an indicator of cardiac output
- **E.** Decreases in air embolism

Q 126. With respect to gas cylinders

- **A.** The maximum pressure in an oxygen cylinder is 4,400 kPa
- **B.** Oxygen cylinders contain liquid and vapour
- **C.** They are made of pure steel
- **D.** Nitrous oxide cylinders contain liquid and vapour
- **E.** The maximum pressure in a nitrous oxide cylinder is 137 bar

Q 127. The following have infrared absorption spectra which overlap with that of carbon dioxide

- **A.** Oxygen
- **B.** Water
- **C.** Nitrous oxide
- **D.** Halothane
- **E.** Helium

Q 128. In a typical blood gas analyser

    A. Oxygen tension will be overestimated in hypothermia
    B. pH is a derived measurement
    C. Standard bicarbonate can be used to indicate the respiratory component
    D. The oxygen tension can be measured using a Clarke electrode
    E. pH value will be raised by the presence of heparin

Q 129. A desflurane vapouriser

    A. Requires heating because desflurane is not volatile
    B. Is pressurised
    C. Runs at $37°C$
    D. Produces a SVP of 1,550 mmHg
    E. Needs a battery backup

Q 130. Gas chromatography

    A. Involves a carrier gas
    B. Involves electron capture as a detector
    C. Uses flame ionisation as a detector
    D. Temperature is maintained constant
    E. Uses a katharometer as a detector

Q 131. The following are agent-specific

    A. Mass spectrometry
    B. IR analysis
    C. UV analysis
    D. Density
    E. Refractive index

Q 132. Refractometers

    A. Are capable of measuring vapour concentration in gas mixture
    B. Require calibration
    C. Directly measure the vapour concentration
    D. Are not influenced by water vapour
    E. Are used to calibrate vapourisers

Q 133. Halothane can be measured by

    A. Raman scattering
    B. Absorption in infrared light
    C. Absorption of ultra-violet light
    D. Mass spectrometry
    E. Solubility in rubber

Q 134. Defibrillators

    A. Contain a capacitor which charges to 4,000 V
    B. Discharge in an exponential manner
    C. Deliver the charge as that which is stored
    D. Thoracic impedance reduces after the first shock
    E. Contain an inductor in the circuit to reduce current duration

Q 135. A Rubens valve

    A. Is a pressure reducing valve
    B. Employs a bobbin and spring system
    C. Will not allow spontaneous respiration
    D. May jam in the expiratory position
    E. Is a non-rebreathing valve

Q 136. Entonox

    A. Is stored in cylinders as a liquid
    B. Should be stored above 10°C
    C. Is a 50:50 mixture of N_2O and oxygen
    D. Has a filling ratio of 0.5
    E. Is stored at 137 bar

Q 137. Entonox

    A. Separates if the cylinder is cooled below 7°C
    B. Cylinders are blue with black and white shoulders
    C. Is stored at 400 kPa
    D. Should be stored upright
    E. Exhibits the Poynting effect

Q 138. Soda lime

- **A.** Should be used dry
- **B.** Contains potassium hydroxide
- **C.** Should be loosely packed
- **D.** Absorbs carbon dioxide in an adiabatic process
- **E.** Turns from white to pink when exhausted

Q 139. Helium

- **A.** Is a component of air
- **B.** Is very soluble
- **C.** Is supplied in green cylinders
- **D.** Is useful in lower airway obstruction
- **E.** Is available in 50% oxygen as 'heliox'

Q 140. Nitrous oxide

- **A.** Has a critical temperature of 34.5°C
- **B.** Supports combustion
- **C.** Boils at −183°C
- **D.** Is supplied in a cylinder with pin index 3, 5
- **E.** Is manufactured by heating ammonium nitrate

Q 141. High air flow oxygen enriched (HAFOE) devices

- **A.** Use the Bernoulli principle
- **B.** Are variable performance
- **C.** Deliver constant concentrations of oxygen
- **D.** Require oxygen entrainment
- **E.** Require closed face masks

Q 142. Gas cylinders

- **A.** Are made of carbon steel
- **B.** Should have the yoke greased to avoid sticking in an emergency
- **C.** Are tested with a hydraulic ram
- **D.** Carry a stamp with their empty weight
- **E.** Have a specific pin index system

Q 143. The following are correct pipeline pressures

    A. Oxygen = 4 bar
    B. Carbon dioxide = 4 bar
    C. Air = 7 bar
    D. Nitrous oxide = 4 bar
    E. Entonox = 7 bar

Q 144. With regard to surgical lasers

    A. The light is monochromatic and the waves are in phase
    B. Argon lasers can be transmitted by optical fibres
    C. They are Class 1 lasers
    D. Carbon dioxide lasers have poor penetration
    E. They are not able to penetrate special laser ET tubes

Q 145. In the Mapleson classification of breathing systems

    A. Mapleson A describes a Lack circuit
    B. Mapleson D is the same as a Magill circuit
    C. Mapleson F is used for paediatric anaesthesia
    D. Mapleson E is the most efficient system for spontaneous respiration
    E. Ayre's T Piece is a Mapleson F circuit

Q 146. The Magill circuit

    A. Is efficient for spontaneous breathing
    B. Is efficient for controlled ventilation
    C. Is appropriate for all ages
    D. Requires a FGF of 2.5 times minute ventilation for spontaneous breathing
    E. Is available in coaxial versions

Q 147. Time-cycled pressure generators

    A. Use a driving gas at 4 bar
    B. Produce an exponential inspiratory flow
    C. Peak pressure relates to airway resistance
    D. Changes in compliance affect tidal volume
    E. Do not compensate for small leaks

Q 148. In soda lime

A. The main constituent is sodium hydroxide
B. Water is required for it to work
C. The carbon dioxide absorbed produces water
D. 1% potassium hydroxide is added to provide a hardening agent
E. The reaction is endothermic

Q 149. Electroencephalograms

A. Vary between 1 and 10 μV
B. Have an alpha band between 4 and 13 Hz
C. Have a theta band between 4–7 Hz
D. Increase in signal amplitude under anaesthesia
E. Are used in the cerebral function analysing monitor

Q 150. Laminar flow of a fluid through a tube is directly related to

A. Length of the tube
B. Viscosity of the fluid
C. Density of the fluid
D. The square of the radius of the tube
E. The pressure difference across the length of the tube

Q 1. **Signs of increasing intracranial pressure may include**

    A. Decreasing level of consciousness
    B. Hypotension
    C. Small pupils
    D. Tachycardia
    E. Rhinorrhoea

Q 2. **Which of the following are correct**

    A. Vagus nerve innervates the epiglottis
    B. Recurrent laryngeal nerve gives the motor supply to the abductors of the vocal cords
    C. Median nerve supplies the outer 3½ fingers
    D. Subclavian vein is posterior to the artery
    E. Subarachnoid space ends at L2

Q 3. **In a patient with a recent head injury the following are indications for immediate surgery**

    A. Depressed skull fracture
    B. Extradural haematoma
    C. Subdural haematoma
    D. CSF rhinorrhoea
    E. Hydrocephalus

Q 4. **DC cardioversion may be indicated in**

    A. Ventricular tachycardia
    B. Premature atrial contractions
    C. Atrial flutter
    D. Digitalis toxicity
    E. Supraventricular tachycardia

Q 5. **Which of the following nerves supply the intrinsic muscles of the larynx**

- **A.** Internal laryngeal
- **B.** Hypoglossal
- **C.** Those originating in the nucleus ambiguus
- **D.** Recurrent laryngeal
- **E.** Glossopharyngeal

Q 6. **Deep venous thrombosis (DVT) is more common in**

- **A.** Elderly patients
- **B.** Patients with malignant disease
- **C.** Patients with cardiac failure
- **D.** Patients receiving dextrans
- **E.** Patients on hormone replacement therapy

Q 7. **The following ECG changes are seen with hyperkalaemia**

- **A.** Loss of p wave
- **B.** Widening of QRS
- **C.** VF
- **D.** Increased size of T wave
- **E.** Increased size of U wave

Q 8. **In a pressure cycled ventilator**

- **A.** The cycling pressure is determined by the patients compliance
- **B.** The inspiratory time is fixed
- **C.** It is a minute volume divider
- **D.** The expiratory period may be time cycled
- **E.** The tidal volume is fixed

Q 9. **Regarding statistics**

- **A.** The middle observation in an ordered series is a median
- **B.** The mean is the most frequently occurring observation in a series
- **C.** Standard deviation gives an indication of the scatter of observations

D. 95% of all observations should lie within ± 2 standard deviations

E. Standard deviation is a measure of the significance of observations

✓ Q 10. Regarding statistics

A. The standard deviation is the square root of the variance

B. The standard deviation is less than the standard error

C. A type I error occurs when the null hypothesis is rejected when it is true

D. The power of a study is defined as $1-$ type II error rate

E. The student's t test can be applied to normally distributed data

Q 11. Features of fat embolism syndrome include

A. Fat in the sputum

B. Fat in the urine

C. Petechial haemorrhages

D. Apyrexia

E. Eye changes

Q 12. The femoral nerve

A. Is included in the '3 in 1' block

B. Gives off a branch to the skin of the scrotum

C. Lies medial to the femoral vein

D. Lies within the femoral sheath with artery, vein and lymph node.

E. When blocked provides suitable anaesthesia for reduction of a fractured neck of femur

Q 13. Signs of adequate reversal of neuromuscular blockade include

A. Sustained head lift for 5 s

B. Good tidal volume

C. Normal arterial carbon dioxide

D. Adequate minute volume

E. Train-of-four ratio greater than 70%

Q 14. Measures to decrease the incidence of suxamethonium pains include

- **A.** A small dose of suxamethonium pre-induction
- **B.** A small dose of non-depolarising muscle relaxant pre-induction
- **C.** Dantrolene 2 h pre-operatively
- **D.** Concurrent intravenous fentanyl
- **E.** Exercise prior to induction

Q 15. Headache following spinal anaesthesia

- **A.** Usually lasts longer than 24 h
- **B.** Is more likely if a 22 G needle is used rather than 26 G
- **C.** Is due to raised CSF pressure
- **D.** Is associated with VIth nerve palsy
- **E.** Can be treated with an epidural blood patch

Q 16. Immediate treatment of anaphylaxis includes

- **A.** Corticosteroid administration
- **B.** 0.5 mg adrenaline i.v.
- **C.** Oxygen
- **D.** Prochlorperazine i.m.
- **E.** Aminophylline i.v.

Q 17. Mendelson's syndrome is associated with

- **A.** Pulmonary oedema
- **B.** Urticarial rash
- **C.** Bronchospasm
- **D.** Cyanosis
- **E.** Methaemoglobinaemia

Q 18. The following are reduced in the elderly patient

- **A.** Functional residual capacity (FRC)
- **B.** Arterial oxygen tension
- **C.** Alveolar oxygen tension
- **D.** Forced expiratory volume
- **E.** MAC of halothane

Q 19. The following factors increase the risk of DVT

- **A.** Obesity
- **B.** Polycythaemia
- **C.** Malignancy
- **D.** Heparin
- **E.** Nephrotic syndrome

Q 20. The following statements apply to day case anaesthesia

- **A.** ASA III patients are not suitable
- **B.** Driving may be permitted within 24 h
- **C.** Starvation is not mandatory
- **D.** Intubation is acceptable
- **E.** All cases should be seen by the anaesthetist before discharge

Q 21. Complications of supraclavicular brachial plexus block include

- **A.** Pneumothorax
- **B.** Horner's syndrome
- **C.** Ptosis
- **D.** Convulsions
- **E.** Phrenic nerve damage

Q 22. The following factors affect minimum alveolar concentration (MAC) value

- **A.** Premedication
- **B.** Age
- **C.** Altitude
- **D.** Agent
- **E.** Sympathetic stimulation

Q 23. With respect to the scavenging of gases and vapours

- **A.** A large pressure gradient is used
- **B.** Scavenging is always passive
- **C.** Sub-atmospheric pressures are used
- **D.** A pressure relief valve is required
- **E.** Passive systems are affected by wind

Q 24. With regard to cardiopulmonary resuscitation (CPR)

A. Survival is more likely if the rhythm is ventricular fibrillation
B. Chest compressions should be 100/min
C. For two resuscitators the ventilation/compression ratio should be 10:1
D. For a single resuscitator the ventilation/compression ratio should be 15:2
E. The approximate tidal volume for a rescue breath without supplemental oxygen is 500 ml

Q 25. In disseminated intravascular coagulation (DIC)

A. Gram-negative septicaemia is a predisposing factor
B. Fibrinolysis is reduced
C. Heparin is contraindicated
D. Thrombocytopenia occurs
E. Treatment with fresh frozen plasma is appropriate

Q 26. With respect to gas/air embolism

A. Up to 30% of the population have a potentially patent foramen ovale
B. Risk factors include positive pressure ventilation
C. A classical sign is the presence of a machinery murmur
D. End-tidal carbon dioxide ($ETCO_2$) may suddenly rise
E. Management includes placing the patient in the head down and left lateral position

Q 27. In rapid sequence induction

A. Non-depolarising relaxants are used
B. Cricoid pressure of 30 N is required
C. Opioids are contraindicated
D. Pre-oxygenation with five vital capacity breaths is adequate
E. Failure of the jaw to relax following suxamethonium may necessitate a second dose.

Q 28. Drugs which trigger malignant hyperpyrexia include

A. Suxamethonium
B. Pancuronium

C. Lidocaine

D. Thiopentone

E. Halothane

Q 29. A patient who cannot breathe 1h after 50mg of suxamethonium may

A. Have homozygous atypical gene for plasma cholinesterase

B. Have malignant hyperpyrexia

C. Have liver disease

D. Require stored blood to raise plasma cholinesterase

E. Require intravenous cholinesterase

Q 30. With regard to local anaesthesia for foot surgery

A. Nerves blocked in an ankle block include tibial, sural, deep and superficial peroneal nerves and saphenous nerve

B. The sural nerve is a branch of the tibial nerve

C. Complete anaesthesia of the foot can be obtained following popliteal nerve block at the knee

D. The saphenous nerve supplies sensation to the ventral aspect of the foot

E. The saphenous nerve may be blocked at the knee

Q 31. The femoral nerve

A. Lies medial to the femoral artery

B. May supply part of the foot

C. Successful block only requires 5 ml of local anaesthetic

D. Block is suitable for malleolar surgery

E. Block is suitable for knee surgery

Q 32. In a patient with a permanent pacemaker in situ presenting for total hip replacement

A. The first letter of the 5 letter code indicates the paced chamber

B. Unipolar diathermy should never be used

C. If the patient has an automated defibrillator function programmed it should be turned off immediately before anaesthesia

D. If DC shock is required intraoperatively the paddles should be placed parallel to the direction of the pacing wire to avoid damaging it

E. External pacing electrodes should be placed over the cardiac apex anteriorly and under the tip of the scapula posteriorly

Q 33. Inadequate depth of anaesthesia leads to

A. Lacrimation

B. Regular respiration

C. Mydriasis

D. Hypertension

E. Bradycardia

Q 34. Clinical features of pneumothorax include

A. Chest pain

B. Breathlessness

C. Productive cough

D. Dull percussion note

E. Reduced breath sounds

Q 35. Malignant hyperthermia (MH)

A. Is inherited as an autosomal dominant condition

B. Is often linked to the ryanodine receptor on chromosome 18

C. May be triggered by nitrous oxide

D. Most patients presenting with MH have had a previous uneventful anaesthetic

E. Results in early, rapid temperature rise

Q 36. Difficulty in intubation will be increased by

A. Increase in posterior depth of the mandible

B. Increased alveolar-mental distance

C. Receding incisors

D. Temporomandibular joint fibrosis

E. Increased distance from the C1 spinous process to the occiput

Q 37. With respect to disinfection/sterilisation of medical equipment

A. Disinfection kills most organisms but not spores
B. Ethylene oxide results in sterilisation
C. Spores are killed by 2% gluteraldehyde
D. Pasteurisation occurs after 5 min at 100°C
E. Sterilisation can be achieved using dry heat at 120°C for 30 min

Q 38. Concerning carbon monoxide poisoning

A. Compared with oxygen, carbon monoxide has 250 times the affinity for the beta chain of the haemoglobin molecule
B. Symptoms include headache, nausea and vomiting
C. Criteria for hypebaric oxygen therapy includes an HBO level >20%
D. The half-life of COHb in air is 2–3 h
E. The half-life of COHb in 100% oxygen at 1 atmosphere is 40–80 min

Q 39. The inguinal canal

A. Extends from the internal ring medially to the external ring laterally
B. The anterior wall is formed by the inguinal ligament
C. Contains the round ligament of the uterus
D. Contains the iliohypogastric nerve
E. Spermatic cord contains autonomic nerve fibres

Q 40. With respect to the larynx

A. The recurrent laryngeal nerve is sensory to the mucosa above the cords
B. The external laryngeal nerve supplies the cricothyroid muscle
C. The recurrent laryngeal nerve carries abductor and adductor fibres
D. The blood supply arises from branches of the superior and inferior thyroid arteries
E. Single cord paralysis requires surgery

Q 41. Damage to the following nerves can occur with incorrect positioning in the lithotomy position

A. Sciatic
B. Lateral popliteal
C. Saphenous
D. Obturator
E. Femoral

Q 42. The following occur after massive transfusion of citrated blood

A. Metabolic acidosis
B. Decreased plasma ionised calcium
C. Hypokalaemia
D. Hyponatraemia
E. Hypothermia

Q 43. Features of pure mitral stenosis on a chest X-ray include

A. A prominent right heart border
B. Splaying of the carina
C. Cardiomegaly
D. Kerley B lines
E. 'Pruning' of peripheral pulmonary vessels

Q 44. The trigeminal nerve supplies

A. The mucosa of the soft palate
B. The tympanic membrane
C. The skin over the angle of the mandible
D. The ala nasae
E. The conjunctiva

Q 45. Regarding latex allergy

A. Premedication is essential in patients suspected of having latex allergy
B. Allergic reactions begin immediately on contact
C. There is an increased incidence in patients with spina bifida
D. There is an increased risk in patients known to be sensitive to bananas
E. Anaphylaxis is a type IV hypersensitivity reaction

Q 46. Regarding the blood supply of the heart

A. The right coronary artery runs in the anterior atrio-ventricular groove

B. The coronary sinus is in the anterior atrio-ventricular groove

C. The venae cordi minimi (Thebesian veins) drain directly into the cardiac chambers

D. There are no anastamoses between the right and left coronary circulations

E. The atrio-ventricular node is supplied by the left coronary artery

Q 47. Regarding sickle cell disease (SCD)

A. Sickle cell – Haemoglobin C (SC) disease has a less severe clinical course

B. Patients may have hyposplenism

C. Most pain is usually easily treated with NSAIDs and paracetamol

D. Alcohol may precipitate a sickle crisis

E. HbS has lysine instead of glutamic acid at position 6 of the alpha chain

Q 48. The epidural space

A. Is a closed space

B. Lies between the spinal dura mater and the arachnoid mater

C. Continues through the foramen magnum into the skull

D. Ends at about the second sacral segment

E. Contains veins whose valves direct flow into the azygos system

Q 49. In acute intermittent porphyria (AIP)

A. Diagnosis is by finding aminolaevulinic acid (ALA) in the urine

B. Treatment may include intravenous haematin

C. Carbohydrates should be avoided

D. Chest symptoms are the commonest to present

E. The inheritance is autosomal dominant

Q 50. Haemolysis, elevated liver enzymes and low platelets (HELLP) syndrome in pregnancy may cause

A. Arterial hypotension
B. Jaundice
C. Haemolytic anaemia
D. Hypoglycaemia
E. Polyuria

Q 1.   The knee jerk

A. Is a monosynaptic reflex
B. Arises from the spinal cord at T12
C. Afferents are from the quadriceps tendon
D. Is not affected by higher centres
E. Afferents come from the quadriceps muscle

Q 2.   Which of the following are true

A. Vertebrate myelinated nerve fibres are between 1 and 20 microns in diameter
B. When a nerve impulse reaches the muscle 'end-plate' electrical transmission occurs
C. 5-hydroxytryptamine is one of the neurotransmitters at the skeletal neuromuscular junction
D. The motor neurones running to intrafusal fibres are gamma-motor fibres
E. Fusimotor nerves are afferent only

Q 3.   The vesicles in the adrenal medulla

A. Contain isoprenaline
B. Store catecholamines and chromogranins
C. Contain DOPA decarboxylase
D. Calcium ions are involved in the release process
E. Release is cholinergic

Q 4.   The conduction velocity along a nerve

A. Increases with diameter
B. Is increased by myelination
C. Increases when the serum potassium is low
D. Is greater in motor than in sensory nerves
E. Is greater in delta than in alpha fibres

Q 5. **The following are transmitters at autonomic ganglia**

A. Dopamine

B. Metacholine

C. GABA

D. 5-HT

E. Glycine

Q 6. **Nerve fibres**

A. Have a lower electrical resistance than surrounding body fluids and tissues

B. The velocity of propagation of the impulse is faster in larger fibres

C. The fastest conduction velocities are about 100 m/s

D. Pain fibres are unmyelinated and are A-delta and C-fibres

E. Smaller fibres are less susceptible to local anaesthetics

Q 7. **These modalities correspond to their pathways**

A. Proprioception via the dorsal columns

B. Temperature and pain via the contralateral spinothalamic tracts

C. Fibres subserving fine touch form the gracile and cuneate nuclei

D. Proprioception and the pyramidal tract

E. Spinocerebellar tracts cross before reaching the cerebellum

Q 8. **Muscle spindles**

A. Are the receptors which excite the normal reflex arc

B. Carry afferent impulses in fusimotor fibres

C. Respond to a rise in muscle tension either from contraction or external stretch

D. Are bundles of modified intrafusal fibres equipped with sensory and motor nerves

E. Are found in smooth muscle

Q 9. **The membrane potential of a nerve fibre**

A. Represents an imbalance of charge across the two sides of a semi-permeable membrane

B. Can be calculated from the Nernst equation

C. Is inversely related to the diameter of the fibre
D. Is measured conventionally as negative on the inside
E. Reverses its polarity during an action potential

Q 10. The non-specialised cell membrane is

A. Permeable to ionic cations
B. Freely permeable to water
C. Permeable to nitrogen
D. Freely permeable to glucose
E. Poorly penetrated by hydrophobic molecules

Q 11. The nerve action potential

A. Is initiated by potassium efflux
B. Is propagated exponentially
C. Transmission is 'saltatory' between the nodes of Ranvier
D. Is conducted faster in myelinated fibres
E. Is approximately 50 mV above the resting potential

Q 12. Cerebrospinal fluid (CSF)

A. 70% is produced by the choroid plexuses within the cerebral ventricles
B. pH is alkaline relative to serum
C. Total volume is about 150 ml
D. Contains 70 g/l protein
E. Is iso-osmolar with plasma

Q 13. Lymph

A. Has a higher protein content than plasma
B. Is produced in a volume of 6 l per 24 h period
C. Has a lipid transport function
D. Contains all coagulation factors
E. Contains platelets in abundance

Q 14. The autonomic nervous system (ANS)

A. Is independent of conscious control
B. Is the efferent pathway to viscera
C. Parasympathetic fibres arise from roots T1–L2

Physiology

Questions

D. Transmits visceral sensation

E. The main sympathetic outflow is from the cranial and sacral regions

Q 15. Pain

A. Transmission normally occurs in the corticospinal tracts

B. May be modulated at a spinal level by peptidergic interneurones

C. Is modified at a spinal level by descending fibres from the periaqueductal grey matter of the mid-brain

D. Is integrated in the thalamus

E. Fibres terminate in the cord in laminae VII–X

Q 16. Intraocular pressure (IOP)

A. Is directly proportional to the blood pressure

B. Is increased by coughing

C. Is reduced by hyperventilation

D. Depends on the angle of the anterior chamber

E. Is unaffected by posture

Q 17. The withdrawal reflex

A. Is a polysynaptic reflex

B. Can be demonstrated by stretching a muscle beyond the length at which the stretch reflex is exhibited

C. As the stimulus increases more limbs will be involved in the response

D. Is unaffected by higher centres

E. Is an example of a mass reflex

Q 18. Autonomic ganglia

A. Adrenaline and acetylcholine are transmitters

B. Autonomic ganglia only exist in the sympathetic nervous system

C. Are linked to the spinal cord by grey rami communicantes

D. Separate pre-and postganglionic fibres

E. White rami communicantes are postganglionic neurones

Q 19. When the nerve cell membrane is suddenly depolarised sodium permeability

A. Falls immediately to zero
B. Falls only slowly remaining low until the membrane potential is restored
C. Rises immediately and is maintained at this level
D. Rises only momentarily
E. Is directly responsible for impulse transmission

Q 20. In the control of body temperature

A. Shivering is a spinal reflex
B. Energy from brown fat is released via adrenergic receptors
C. The thalamus has a role
D. Tumour necrosis factor (TNF) may cause pyrexia
E. Normal temperature is highest in the night

Q 21. With respect to vascular tone

A. It is mediated via an alpha adrenergic effect
B. It is mediated locally by noradrenaline
C. Sympathectomy induces vasodilation
D. Sympathectomy produces no effect on vessel diameter but flow is increased
E. Vasodilatation occurs in response to cold and haemorrhage

Q 22. The following neurotransmitters are correctly associated

A. Acetylcholine and the limbic system
B. Serotonin and the limbic system
C. Dopamine and the thalamus
D. Noradrenaline and the cerebral cortex
E. Noradrenaline and the cerebellum

Q 23. Water intoxication may cause the following

A. Coma
B. Vomiting
C. Hypernatraemia
D. Convulsions
E. Delirium

Q 24. The oxygen content of blood is decreased in

A. COHb
B. Methaemoglobinaemia
C. Anaemia
D. Chronic renal failure
E. Hyperbaric conditions

Q 25. Raised left ventricular end diastolic pressure (LVEDP)

A. Is caused by increased left ventricular compliance
B. Increases myocardial oxygen consumption
C. Occurs commonly in mitral stenosis
D. Results in decreased myocardial work
E. Occurs with aortic regurgitation

Q 26. Iodine

A. Is necessary for thyroxine synthesis
B. Is concentrated in the breast
C. Has no effect on thyroid histology
D. Is added to salt sold in this country
E. Is concentrated in the salivary glands

Q 27. Haemoglobin

A. Contains four alpha chains
B. Carries four molecules of oxygen per chain
C. Is a four-chain structure
D. Contains a ferric ion
E. Is a polysaccharide

Q 28. The knee jerk

A. Is due to stimulation of receptors in the patellar tendon
B. Is propagated through the lumbar segment L2
C. Has a reflex arc which involves a single interneurone
D. Involves the femoral nerve
E. Is abolished immediately after transection of the spinal cord at T6

Q 29. Blood flow in ml per 100 g of tissue is

 A. Brain – 54
 B. Heart – 84
 C. Whole body – 26
 D. Kidneys – 420
 E. Skin – 22

Q 30. Myoglobin

 A. Combines reversibly with oxygen
 B. Has a larger molecular weight than haemoglobin
 C. Acts as a temporary oxygen store in muscles
 D. Does not show the Bohr effect
 E. Combines reversibly with carbon dioxide

Q 31. Carbon dioxide

 A. Is carried on the haemoglobin molecule as carboxyhaemoglobin
 B. In the blood increases the oxygen binding power of haemoglobin
 C. Entry into the blood results in the movement of chloride ions into the erythrocytes
 D. Is carried in dissolved form at 20% of the total
 E. Is less soluble in the blood than oxygen

Q 32. The following factors increase the cardiac output

 A. Sitting or standing from the lying position
 B. Rapid arrhythmias
 C. Eating
 D. Exercise
 E. Hypothermia

Q 33. A shift of the oxygen haemoglobin dissociation curve to the right

 A. Occurs in the pulmonary capillaries
 B. Is favoured by a rise in temperature
 C. Favours the passage of oxygen from blood to the tissues
 D. Occurs when foetal blood is replaced by adult blood
 E. Is favoured by a decrease in blood pH

Q 34. Gastric emptying is increased by

A. Gastrin
B. Eating a meal containing a large amount of fat
C. Vagotomy
D. Sympathetic stimulation
E. Fat in the duodenum

Q 35. With respect to the heart

A. Atrial contraction is not significant in ventricular filling
B. Ventricular filling does not occur during the phase of isovolumetric ventricular relaxation
C. Coronary blood flow is greatest during diastole
D. Coronary blood flow decreases in response to myocardial hypoxia
E. The bundle of Kent is usually present

Q 36. In the heart

A. Coronary blood flow is 250 ml/min at rest
B. The SA node is innervated by the left vagus
C. The AV node is innervated by the right vagus
D. Stroke volume falls when the vagus is stimulated
E. Stroke volume is independent of the duration of the previous diastole

Q 37. The Fick principle is used to measure

A. Renal output
B. Respiratory rate
C. Cerebral blood flow
D. Cardiac output
E. Peripheral limb blood flow

Q 38. An increase in right atrial pressure

A. Decreases systemic arterial pressure
B. Increases cardiac output
C. Causes an increase in urine volume
D. Can increase the heart rate via the Bainbridge reflex
E. Can decrease the heart rate via the baroreceptor reflex

Q 39. The following usually exist in the normal circulation in the inactivated state

A. Fibrin
B. Thrombin
C. Plasminogen
D. Christmas factor
E. Anti-haemophilic factor

Q 40. In the jugular venous pressure wave

A. Cannon waves occur with atrial contraction against a closed tricuspid valve
B. Tricuspid regurgitation causes early onset and prominent 'v' waves
C. The peak of the 'c' wave occurs in mid-systole
D. In cardiac tamponade there is short steep 'y' descent followed by a sustained elevation in pressure
E. The 'x' descent follows the 'v' wave

Q 41. At birth

A. The foramen ovale closes because of a reversal of the pressure gradient between the left and right atria
B. The ductus arteriosus closes because of a metabolic acidosis
C. The ductus arteriosus closes because of a reversal of the pressure gradient between pulmonary artery and aorta
D. Lung compliance decreases
E. The first breath generates a negative pressure of about 10 cmH$_2$O

Q 42. Immediately after complete transection of the spinal cord the following features may be found below the lesion

A. Loss of motor power but preservation of limb reflexes
B. Urinary incontinence
C. Loss of muscle power but preservation of sensation
D. Flaccid paralysis with loss of limb reflexes
E. Loss of muscle power but preservation of muscle joint position sense

Q 43. Blood transfusion

A. Has an incidence of viral hepatitis of 1% or less
B. Incompatible transfusion will cause a fall in fibrinogen
C. 1 Unit of blood will raise the Hb value by 10% in 24 h
D. May result in pulmonary oedema
E. All blood is tested for *Treponema pallidum*

Q 44. Regarding the maintenance of body pH

A. The bicarbonate buffer system is the most important
B. The normal H^+ concentration in arterial blood is about 40 nmol/l
C. Plasma proteins have more buffering capacity than haemoglobin
D. The pKa for the bicarbonate buffer system is about 6.3
E. The phosphate buffer is important in the extracellular fluid

Q 45. In amniotic fluid embolus the following are seen

A. Respiratory distress
B. Decreased fibrinogen levels
C. Hypoxia
D. Coma
E. Coagulopathy

Q 46. Stimulation of different regions of the hypothalamus could cause effects on

A. Eating
B. Water balance
C. Temperature regulation
D. Sexual activity
E. Blood pressure

Q 47. Concerning gastro-intestinal secretions

A. Saliva has a pH of 4.0
B. Gastric pH may be as low as 1.0
C. Gastric secretions contain intrinsic factor
D. Pancreatic secretions have a pH of greater than 12.5
E. Saliva contains IgA

Q 48. Immediately after complete division of a mixed peripheral nerve

A. The denervated muscles exhibit the characteristic features of an 'upper motor neurone lesion'
B. There is a loss of sensation in the denervated area of skin
C. The denervated area of skin will be cooler than the surrounding area
D. The sweat gland in the denervated area of skin will respond to an increase in temperature of the hypothalamus
E. The cut nerve fibres of the central stump are capable of regeneration along the nerve sheath

Q 49. Consequences of starvation include

A. Increased brain uptake of glucose
B. Reduction of the respiratory quotient
C. Elevated blood glucagon levels
D. Increased urinary nitrogen output
E. Development of metabolic alkalosis

Q 50. Active transport across cell membranes

A. Is increased by hypothermia
B. Transfers hydrogen ions into gastric juice against a concentration gradient
C. Requires energy production by the cell
D. Aids hydrogen ion secretion by the kidney tubule cells
E. Prevents an excess of water from entering the cell

Q 51. The extracellular fluid in man

A. Comprises the interstitial fluid and the blood plasma
B. May be measured by use of the Fick principle
C. May be measured using radioactive potassium
D. Contains most of the magnesium in the body
E. If reduced in volume causes a rise in blood pressure

Q 52. With reference to endocrine function

A. Growth hormone is involved in the control of growth of the long bones during adolescence

B. Cortisol concentration in the plasma exerts a negative feedback effect on hypothalamic production of corticotrophic releasing factor
C. Steroid hormones are normally bound to plasma proteins
D. Adrenal androgens are normally secreted only in the male
E. Release of antidiuretic hormone from the posterior pituitary is increased when osmolality of cerebral extracellular fluid increases

Q 53. In diastolic function

A. Myocardial relaxation is metabolically inactive
B. Catecholamines cause positive lusitropy
C. Atrial contraction contributes up to 40% of ventricular filling in the normal heart
D. The greater part of left coronary artery blood flow occurs
E. Diastasis shortens first with increasing heart rate

Q 54. In the foetal circulation

A. The right ventricle posses a thicker wall than the left
B. The ductus arteriosus closes due to pressure changes
C. There is a lower pO_2 in the descending aorta than in the aortic arch
D. There is a lower pO_2 in the ductus arteriosus than in the ductus venosus
E. Blood can pass through IVC to the aorta without passing through the left atrium or ventricle

Q 55. In the pregnant woman

A. There is reduced red cell mass
B. There is a reduced haematocrit
C. There is a reduced $PaCO_2$
D. There is reduced protein bound iodine
E. Oxygen consumption is reduced

Q 56. In normal spontaneously breathing subject in lateral position

A. Blood flow is highest in the lower lung
B. Ventilation is highest in the lower lung

C. pO_2 is higher in blood from lower lung

D. $PaCO_2$ is higher in blood from lower lung

E. FRC is reduced

Q 57. In the normal subject going from upright to supine

A. There is decreased blood pressure

B. There is decreased pressure in leg veins

C. There is increased venous return

D. There is increased capacity of pulmonary veins

E. Mean arterial pressure (MAP) falls

Q 58. Venous blood from the following tissues have a lower pO_2 than that of mixed venous blood

A. Heart

B. Liver

C. Kidney

D. Brain

E. Resting muscle

Q 59. Acetylcholine is released by

A. Preganglionic sympathetic neurones

B. All postganglionic sympathetic neurones

C. Preganglionic parasympathetic neurones

D. Postganglionic parasympathetic neurones

E. Motor nerves at neuromuscular junction

Q 60. Rate of gastric emptying is

A. Slowed by fat in oesophagus

B. Unaffected by meal size

C. Reduced by carbohydrate in duodenum

D. Reduced by acid in duodenum

E. Increased by secretin

Q 61. Aldosterone

A. Is released following a sodium load

B. Is released following fluid overload

C. Secretion is stimulated by ACTH

D. Release involves renin

E. Causes calcium loss

Q 62. Pain sensation

A. Is carried primarily in the dorsal columns

B. Felt in response to a normally non-painful stimulus is called hyperalgesia

C. May be elicited by direct stimulation of the cerebral cortex

D. May be reduced by sympathetic activity (sympathectomy)

E. May be reduced by simultaneous stimulation of other modalities in the same spinal segment

Q 63. Hypothalamic neurones produce the following

A. Prolactin

B. ADH

C. Growth hormone

D. ACTH

E. TSH

Q 64. Insulin

A. Blocks K^+ entry into cells

B. Promotes protein anabolism

C. Promotes hepatic glycolysis

D. Stimulates glucagon release

E. Promotes fat synthesis and deposition

Q 65. Glucagon

A. Is released by A cells of the pancreatic islets

B. Prevents insulin release

C. Is raised following 24h starvation

D. Stimulates glycogenolysis

E. Increases FFA levels

Q 66. Thyroid hormones

A. Are mainly protein bound

B. Protein bound iodine is a useful measure of thyroxine level

C. Follicular cells contain an iodine pump

D. Carbimazole may cause a goitre

E. Act on intracellular receptors

Q 67. The carotid bodies

A. Are more responsive to pO_2 than O_2 content

B. Are more important in humans than the aortic bodies

C. Are located at the division of the common carotid artery

D. Have chemoreceptor cells

E. Have lower blood flow per mcg tissue than brain

Q 68. Cerebrospinal fluid

A. Is a simple ultrafiltrate of plasma

B. Provides for the greater part of the nutritional requirements of the CNS

C. Has the same glucose concentration as plasma

D. Has a lower specific gravity than plasma

E. Passes from the third ventricle to the cisterna magna via the aqueduct

Q 69. Pulmonary surfactant

A. Increases the surface tension of alveolar fluid

B. Increases the compliance of the lungs

C. Is a mucopolysaccharide

D. Is increased following transient interruption of pulmonary blood flow

E. Is absent from the lungs of a full term infant

Q 70. Repeated expiration against a pressure of 10 cmH₂O

A. Increases pulmonary artery pressure

B. Decreases cardiac output

C. Increases end expiratory lung volume

D. May be used to increase arterial oxygen tension

E. Would be expected to increase central venous pressure

Q 71. Muscles active during forced expiration include

A. The diaphragm

B. External oblique

C. Internal oblique
D. Rectus abdominis
E. Scalenus anterior

Q 72. The sympathetic nervous system supplies

A. Dilator fibres to the bronchial tree
B. The ciliary muscles of the eye
C. The radial muscle of the iris
D. The majority of contractile fibres to the detrusor muscle
E. Constrictor fibres to the smooth muscle of the jejunum

Q 73. Increased gamma motor neurone activity will result in

A. Skeletal muscle relaxation
B. Uterine contraction
C. Vasodilatation
D. Increased tone of voluntary muscles
E. Hyperactive tendon reflexes

Q 74. In a resting nerve fibre

A. Membrane potentials can be calculated from the Nernst equation and sodium concentrations
B. The transmembrane potential is 30 mV
C. The transmembrane chloride flux is passive
D. The intra and extracellular Ca^{2+} concentrations are equal
E. The sodium pump is active

Q 75. The sensation of pain

A. Is conveyed to the ventral and medial parts of the thalamus
B. Is augmented by beta endorphin
C. Can be modified by cutting the spinothalamic tract
D. Can be modified by strenuous exercise
E. Can be modified by non-painful stimuli in the same area

Q 76. Interruption of the cervical sympathetic chain causes

A. Engorgement of the nasal mucosa
B. Enophthalmus
C. Decreased lacrimation

D. Conjunctival vasodilatation

E. Meiosis

Q 77. Concerning liver blood flow

A. Portal venous pressure is less than 20 mmHg

B. 50% is from the hepatic artery

C. Total flow is 1.5 l/min

D. The liver derives 90% of its oxygen needs from the portal supply

E. The oxygen saturation of portal blood is 95%

Q 78. Insulin and growth hormone have directly opposing effects on

A. Fat catabolism

B. Glucose utilisation

C. Fat anabolism

D. Protein anabolism

E. Glycogen production

Q 79. The following influence aldosterone secretion

A. Surgical stress

B. Total sodium intake

C. Renal ischaemia

D. Angiotensin

E. Plasma potassium concentration

Q 80. Parathormone

A. Increases plasma calcium concentration

B. Increases bone resorption of Ca^{2+}

C. Increases urinary phosphate loss

D. Is a polypeptide

E. Causes phosphaturia

Q 81. Carotid body receptors

A. Have a higher blood flow gram for gram than the brain

B. Have baroreceptor activity

C. Respond to changes in oxygen content of the blood

D. Contain glomus cells

E. Are not affected by carotid endarterectomy

Q 82. Acutely reducing the inspired oxygen concentration to 10% at sea level will cause

A. Decreased urinary pH

B. Increased cardiac output

C. Decreased capacity of Hb for oxygen

D. A respiratory alkalosis

E. Increased erythropoietin secretion

Q 83. Concerning foetal physiology

A. Type II pneumocytes produce surfactant from week 21

B. The pO_2 in the descending aorta is less than in the ductus arteriosus

C. Breathing movements are made in utero

D. At birth, flow in the ductus arteriosus reverses because of decreased pulmonary resistance

E. Umbilical arterial blood has a higher pO_2 than umbilical venous blood

Q 84. The following occur during exercise

A. Increased body temperature

B. Increased diastolic pressure

C. Potassium loss

D. Decreased stroke volume

E. Increased renal blood flow

Q 85. Renal blood flow

A. Is one-fifth of cardiac output at rest

B. Is decreased by IPPV

C. Is evenly distributed throughout the kidney

D. Is constant between arterial pressures of 75–160 mmHg

E. Decreases with halothane

Q 86. The oxygen-haemoglobin dissociation curve moves to the right

A. With an increase in temperature

B. When 2,3-DPG levels increase

C. When carbon dioxide concentration increases

D. With an increase in hydrogen ion concentration

E. On exercise

Q 87. Concerning the blood-brain barrier

A. Glucose can cross freely

B. It is part of the meninges

C. Permeability alters if it is inflamed

D. It prevents release of central neurotransmitters into the systemic circulation

E. It is more permeable at birth than in adulthood

Q 88. The jugular venous pulse

A. Has a height which reflects central venous pressure

B. Should be measured with a patient at 30 degrees celsius

C. Has an accentuated 'a' wave in atrial fibrillation

D. Shows giant 'v' waves in tricuspid regurgitation

E. Is normally less than 3 cm above the sternal angle

Q 89. In the Valsalva manoeuvre

A. There is an increase in intrathoracic pressure

B. There is a decrease in heart rate

C. There is an increase in cardiac output

D. Peripheral resistance falls

E. Pulse pressure increases

Q 90. With respect to the jugular venous pulse

A. The 'a' wave is due to ventricular systole

B. The 'c' wave is caused by the bulging of the pulmonary valve during isometric contraction

C. The 'v' wave corresponds to the rise in atrial pressure before the opening of the tricuspid valve

D. Cannon waves are not seen in complete heart block

E. A giant 'a' wave is not seen in complete heart block

Q 91. Compared with plasma, CSF contains

A. More cholesterol

B. More sodium

C. More urea

D. More creatinine

E. A higher pCO_2

Q 92. Carbon dioxide is carried in the blood

A. Mainly as bicarbonate

B. Mainly as carbamino compounds

C. Preferentially by oxyhaemoglobin

D. Mainly in solution

E. Mainly combined with haemoglobin

Q 93. Muscles of inspiration include

A. External intercostals

B. Diaphragm

C. Internal intercostals

D. Rectus abdominus

E. Latissimus dorsi

Q 94. The ankle-jerk reflex is

A. Polysynaptic

B. Initiated by receptors in the achilles tendon

C. Initiated by receptors in the gastrocnemius

D. A response to muscle spindle stimulation

E. Absent in cord transection

Q 95. The following statements apply to the Valsalva manoeuvre

A. Initial arterial pressure rises

B. Heart rate is unchanged

C. Preload is reduced

D. It is followed by an increase in arterial pressure

E. It is defined as a forced expiration against a closed glottis

Q 96. In the normal kidney

A. GFR is the same as RPF

B. RPF is 125 ml/min

C. GFR is 600 ml/min

D. Filtration fraction is 0.25

E. GFR may be measured using inulin

Q 97. In acclimatisation to altitude

A. Respiratory acidosis occurs

B. Red cell 2,3-DPG levels fall

C. Ventilation is increased

D. Erythropoietin secretion rises

E. Haematocrit rises

Q 98. Cerebrospinal fluid

A. Has a higher bicarbonate content than blood

B. Contains IgG

C. Total volume is 70 ml

D. Contains white cells

E. Is static within the central nervous system

Q 99. Chemoreceptors are found in

A. The aortic arch

B. The carotid body

C. The carotid sinus

D. The CNS

E. The aortic body

Q 100. In starvation

A. Muscle glycogen and brain glycogen are replenished by gluconeogenesis

B. Free fatty acid oxidation in the liver, muscle and heart is increased

C. Ketone bodies produced in the liver from free fatty acids can be utilised by brain cells but glucose is still essential

D. Glucose can be formed from fatty acids

E. The odour of the breath is due to ketosis

Q 101. The action potential

A. Is generated by differing ionic concentrations of sodium and potassium

B. A negative potential inside the nerve drives potassium ions to the outside

C. Depolarisation is caused by the transfer of sodium ions across the membrane
D. In the resting state the potential inside the nerve fibre is +85 mV
E. At the peak of the action potential the voltage change is 35 mV

Q 102. The T wave of the ECG occurs

A. At the beginning of the refractory period
B. During atrial systole
C. During ventricular diastole
D. During repolarisation of the ventricle
E. At the time of the first heart sound

Q 103. The following statements are true of alveoli

A. The mean wall thickness is 5 microns
B. The pores of Kohn connect to bronchioles
C. They have a mean diameter of 0.5 mm at FRC
D. Type I cells produce surfactant
E. Type I cells occupy 80% of the surface for gas exchange

Q 104. The peripheral chemoreceptors

A. Are stimulated by a reduction in the content of oxygen in arterial blood
B. Contain dopamine
C. Respond more to CO_2 than the central chemoreceptors
D. Are stimulated by exercise
E. Are supplied by the glossopharyngeal nerve

Q 105. The central chemoreceptors

A. Are largely stimulated by hypoxia
B. Are situated beneath the ventral surface of the medulla
C. Are the major source of the response to hypercapnia
D. Are stimulated more rapidly by a change in arterial CO_2 than the peripheral chemoreceptors
E. Are affected by CSF bicarbonate concentration

Q 106. In a fit adult person, anatomical dead space

- **A.** Increases with increasing lung volumes
- **B.** Decreases with hypoventilation
- **C.** Is least when the neck is flexed and chin is down
- **D.** May be measured by Fowler's method
- **E.** Requires measurement of PECO$_2$ to be calculated by Bohr's method

Q 107. In pregnancy

- **A.** Echocardiography has demonstrated left ventricular hypertrophy by 12 weeks
- **B.** The electrical axis of the heart may be rotated to the left
- **C.** ST segment depression is likely to be clinically significant
- **D.** The SVR remains normal
- **E.** A third heart sound is pathological

Q 108. With regard to myosin and actin

- **A.** A myosin molecule has a molecular weight of 80,000 daltons
- **B.** Myosin heads form cross bridges with actin filaments
- **C.** The myosin head acts as an ATPase enzyme
- **D.** Actin filaments are inserted in Z discs
- **E.** ADP molecules are the active sites on actin filaments

Q 109. The following statements apply to liver blood flow

- **A.** The liver receives blood from both systemic and portal circulations
- **B.** It comprises 30% of cardiac output
- **C.** It is 1,500 ml/min
- **D.** Regulation is by local factors
- **E.** Regulation is by the parasympathetic nervous system

Q 110. The following are suitable features of a substance for the measurement of GFR

- **A.** Tubular reabsorption
- **B.** No metabolism
- **C.** No effect on GFR

D. Free filtration
E. Non-toxic

Q 111. The following statements apply to clearance

A. It is defined as the amount of plasma cleared of a substance in unit time
B. Normal creatine clearance is 125 ml/kg/min
C. Inulin clearance measures GFR
D. PAH clearance measures RPF
E. The value of GFR varies greatly during the day

Q 112. The extracellular fluid

A. Volume may be measured with inulin
B. Volume may be measured with mannitol
C. Comprises 50% of body weight
D. Is 20l in the adult
E. Decreases with age when expressed as an index of body surface area

Q 113. Regarding reabsorption of glucose in the kidney

A. The tubular maximum for glucose is relatively independent of endocrine function
B. The tubular maximum is dependent on the blood glucose level
C. The tubular maximum is about 375 mg/min
D. Most reabsorption occurs in the distal tubule
E. The tubular maximum is not homogeneous between nephrons

Q 114. With respect to pain transmissions

A. Fast pain travels in A delta fibres
B. Pain is associated with the ventral spinothalamic tract
C. Descending tracts modulate pain transmission
D. The pain gate lies in the dorsal horn of the spinal cord
E. Slow pain travels in C fibres

Q 115. The oxygen haemoglobin dissociation curve

    A. Will shift to the left in hypothermia
    B. Has a P50 of 3.5 kPa
    C. Has a sigmoid shape
    D. Will shift to the right if 2,3-DPG is reduced
    E. Is affected by carbon monoxide

Q 116. In transfusion medicine

    A. Blood group AB is the rarest in the UK
    B. Patients who are blood group O have IgM antibodies to A and B
    C. Rhesus antibodies are IgM
    D. Kell and Duffy antibodies can cause immediate haemolytic transfusion reactions
    E. Only 10% of individuals secrete ABO substances in their saliva

Q 117. Cardiac output

    A. Increases in moderate exercise mainly due to an increased stroke volume
    B. May be measured by the Fick method
    C. Increases with a rise in pCO_2
    D. May increase up to 15 times in a trained athlete
    E. Falls when IPPV is started

Q 118. The components of vital capacity include

    A. Functional residual capacity
    B. Tidal volume
    C. Residual volume
    D. Inspiratory reserve volume
    E. Expiratory reserve volume

Q 119. In the normal kidney

    A. GFR may be estimated by PAH clearance
    B. Renal plasma flow is around 400 ml/min
    C. The tubular maximum for glucose is 375 mg/min

D. Sodium reabsorption is always passive

E. Urinary pH lies between 3 and 10

Q 120. The carotid body responds to

A. A fall in pH

B. Increased pCO_2

C. A fall in blood pressure

D. Doxapram

E. Increased frequency of impulses in Hering's nerves

Q 121. The transmission of pain

A. Occurs via the spinothalamic tracts

B. Arises from nociceptors

C. Involves peptide neurotransmitters in the substantia gelatinosa

D. Can be initiated by bradykinin

E. Due to cold is initiated by purinergic receptors

Q 122. Function of the liver include

A. Manufacture of plasma proteins

B. Secretion of bile

C. Gluconeogenesis

D. Manufacture of antibodies

E. Acetylation

Q 123. In the first 24 h after major injury

A. Sodium is retained

B. Potassium is lost

C. Metabolic rate is increased

D. Urinary nitrogen levels will fall

E. Glucagon secretion is decreased

Q 124. The pituitary gland secretes

A. Prolactin

B. Corticotrophin releasing factor

C. FSH

D. Long acting thyroid stimulator

E. Vasopressin

Q 125. **The following are muscles of expiration**

    A. Diaphragm
    B. Internal intercostals
    C. External intercostals
    D. Rectus abdominus
    E. Scalenus anterior

Q 126. **Coronary artery blood flow**

    A. Has diastolic pressure as its main determinant
    B. Is unaffected by changes in arterial pressure
    C. Is under some humoral control
    D. Is reduced in severe tachycardia
    E. At rest is about 500 ml/min

Q 127. **Hypomagnesaemia**

    A. Is characterised by muscle weakness
    B. May cause cardiac arrhythmias
    C. May cause convulsions
    D. Is a complication of aminoglycoside therapy
    E. Is usually associated with hypercalcaemia

Q 128. **Cerebral blood flow**

    A. Exhibits large regional variations
    B. Is greater than coronary artery blood flow
    C. Is more susceptible to changes in pO_2 than pCO_2
    D. Is subject to autoregulation
    E. Is affected by local release of metabolites

Q 129. **Peripheral resistance is increased in**

    A. Haemorrhage
    B. Changing from supine to standing
    C. Exercise
    D. Valsalva manoeuvre
    E. High ambient temperature

Q 130. **The non-respiratory functions of the lung include**

    A. Metabolism of dopamine
    B. Metabolism of bradykinin

C. Metabolism of serotonin
D. Production of prostaglandin E2
E. Conversion of angiotensin 1

Q 131. In comparing intracellular contents versus extracellular there is more

A. Phosphate
B. Magnesium
C. ATP
D. Chloride
E. Sodium

Q 132. Anti-diuretic hormone

A. Is the main determinant of whether urine will be copious or dilute
B. Makes the collecting tubules impermeable to urea
C. Needs the presence of cortisol to exert its maximum effect
D. Does not affect water reabsorption in the proximal tubule
E. Is synthesised in the posterior pituitary

Q 133. The following are common to both intrinsic and extrinsic clotting pathways

A. Factor VII
B. Factor V
C. Factor VIII
D. Factor IX
E. Calcium

Q 134. The following stimulate insulin secretion

A. Beta-blockers
B. Glucagon
C. Volatile agents
D. Thiazides
E. Increased amino acid concentrations

Q 135. Active reabsorption of glucose occurs in the

A. Proximal tubules
B. Loops of Henle

C. Distal tubules
D. Collecting ducts
E. Bladder

Q 136. In acclimatisation to altitude

A. Initially hyperventilation occurs
B. The oxygen haemoglobin dissociation curve shifts to the right
C. Erythropoietin secretion increases
D. Tissue content of cytochrome oxidase is increased
E. P50 is increased

Q 137. Basal metabolic rate

A. Is 3,000 kcal/24 h for a 70 kg man
B. Is increased by anxiety
C. Is increased by 20% for each degree Celcius rise in temperature
D. Falls in starvation
E. Is higher in the tropics

Q 138. Myocardial contractility

A. May be defined as the mechanical work performed when it contracts with a pre-defined load and initial degree of stretch
B. Is affected by preload
C. Is inhibited by an increase in intracellular calcium
D. Depends on Starling's law
E. Is affected by heart rate

Q 139. The following are determinants of cardiac output

A. Heart rate
B. Stroke volume
C. Preload
D. Afterload
E. Sympathetic stimulation

Q 140. In complete cord transection

A. Hyperreflexia occurs initially
B. Arterial blood pressure will not change

C. New nerve endings may sprout in the cord

D. Autonomic hyperreflexia occurs within the first few days

E. Bladder control remains throughout

Q 141. Concerning cerebral blood flow

A. It is equally divided between internal carotid and vertebral arteries

B. Blood flow in the white matter may be 4 times that in the grey matter

C. It is equal to 30% of cardiac output

D. It changes approximately 5 ml/100 g/min per mmHg change in pCO_2

E. It is significantly reduced by intracranial pressure over 33 mmHg

Q 142. Regarding haemoglobin

A. It has a molecular weight of 30,000

B. In the foetus it is composed of two alpha and two gamma chains

C. 2,3-DPG is an intermediate metabolite of the citric acid cycle

D. 2,3-DPG binds to the de-oxygenated form

E. The binding of oxygen is 'cooperative'

Q 143. The following are true of sickle cell trait

A. It is a homozygous state

B. It is present in 8–10% of black Americans

C. It presents with severe anaemia

D. It will be detected by the Sickledex test

E. It may be diagnosed by electrophoresis

Q 144. In pregnancy

A. Plasma fibrinogen concentration increases

B. The increase in cardiac output is by increased stroke volume only

C. The cardiac output increases by about 50% overall

D. The functional residual capacity is reduced

E. The residual volume increases

Q 145. Pulmonary vascular resistance

A. Is lowest at FRC
B. Is decreased with increased sympathetic tone
C. Is increased by IPPV
D. Is high in the foetus due to the reduced blood flow through the lungs
E. Is increased at altitude

Q 146. The pain of uterine contraction in labour

A. Passes via the nervi erigentes from the cervix
B. Passes from the body of the uterus via the lumbar sympathetic chain
C. Is perceived in the lower thoracic dermatomes
D. Is transmitted via the lower thoracic nerve roots
E. Is transmitted from the body of the uterus via the cervical plexus

Q 147. Concerning the oxygen-haemoglobin dissociation curve

A. The P50 is the partial pressure of oxygen at which haemoglobin is 50% saturated
B. It lies to the left of the O_2-myoglobin dissociation curve
C. The sigmoid shape is due to cooperative binding
D. If the P50 is increased this represents an increase in the oxygen affinity of haemoglobin
E. It is moved to the left in stored blood

Q 148. In the foetal circulation

A. The pulmonary vascular resistance falls at birth
B. The right atrial pressure is higher than the left
C. Right atrial anatomy preferentially directs blood flow from the SVC through the foramen ovale
D. All blood from the umbilical vein drains directly into the inferior vena cava
E. Pulmonary capillaries are formed prior to 20 weeks gestation

Q 149. The closing capacity

A. Is the lung volume at which airway collapse and closure occurs during expiration

B. Is the same as the closing volume

C. Cannot be measured unless the subject is awake and cooperative

D. May be measured using a vital capacity breath of 100% oxygen

E. Is less than the functional residual capacity in a young adult

Q 150. Cerebral blood flow (CBF)

A. A decrease in arterial pressure causes vasoconstriction of cerebral vessels

B. An increased pH causes vasodilatation

C. A high pO_2 causes cerebral vasoconstriction

D. The normal jugular venous saturation is 40%

E. Can be measured by doppler

Q 1. Adrenaline

A. Is synthesised from noradrenaline by a methyl transferase in the adrenal medulla and nerve endings

B. Increases the basal metabolic rate

C. Is metabolised in the liver

D. Stimulates glycogenolysis

E. Causes systolic and diastolic hypertension when injected intravenously

Q 2. Prostaglandins E2 and F2 are

A. Not naturally occurring substances

B. Used to induce abortion and labour

C. Metabolised in the pulmonary circulation

D. Modulators of histamine and bradykinin action in pain

E. Stored in mast cells

Q 3. Alpha-adrenergic stimulation produces

A. Vasodilation

B. Tachycardia

C. Uterine relaxation

D. A positive inotropic effect

E. Intestinal relaxation

Q 4. Ringer lactate contains (in mmol/l)

A. Na – 131

B. K – 5.0

C. Ca – 4.0

D. Lactate – 29

E. Cl – 112

Q 5. Digitalis toxicity

A. May be indicated by bradycardia and a prolonged P-R interval

B. May be indicated by a supra ventricular tachycardia or ventricular extrasystoles

C. May be reduced by giving calcium salts

D. Is usefully treated by the slow infusion of phenytoin

E. Is an absolute contraindication to beta-blockade

Q 6. Side effects of steroid therapy include

A. Growth retardation in children

B. Osteomalacia

C. Precipitation of diabetes mellitus

D. Glaucoma

E. Depression

Q 7. The rate at which the alveolar concentration of an anaesthetic approaches inspired concentration is a function of

A. Alveolar ventilation

B. Water solubility of agent

C. Cardiac output

D. Saturated vapour pressure

E. Inspired concentration

Q 8. Acetylcholinesterase

A. Is found in plasma

B. Is inhibited by pilocarpine

C. Will hydrolyse dibucaine

D. Hydrolyses acetylcholine faster than other choline esters

E. Is present in high concentration in the placenta

Q 9. Paracetamol

A. Inhibits prostaglandin synthesis

B. Is highly protein bound

C. Has a low bioavailability due to first pass metabolism

D. Can cause thrombocytopaenia at therapeutic levels

E. Is conjugated in the liver to both glucuronide and sulphate conjugates

Q 10. Boiling points

A. Diethyl ether = 104.6°C
B. Cyclopropane = −33°C
C. Nitrous oxide = −88°C
D. Halothane = 50.2°C
E. Trichloroethylene = 34°C

Q 11. Side effects of phenytoin are

A. Ataxia
B. Megaloblastic anaemia
C. Hepatic damage
D. Skin rashes
E. Agranulocytosis

Q 12. In the metabolism of morphine the following mechanisms are used

A. N-dealkylation
B. Glucuronide formation
C. Acetylation
D. Hydrolysis of ester-linkage
E. Oxidative deamination

Q 13. Monoamine oxidase inhibitors

A. Produce mental excitement with methyldopa
B. Can produce cerebellar dysfunction
C. Unlike other antidepressants do not have autonomic disturbances
D. React with the substance tyrosine, which is found in cheese
E. Can be safely used with pentazocine (Fortral)

Q 14. Isoflurane

A. Is a respiratory depressant
B. Is metabolised to inorganic fluoride ions
C. Has been implicated in the causation of seizures
D. Is a structural isomer of halothane
E. Causes a tachycardia

Q 15. Bupivacaine

    A. Is <20% excreted unchanged in the urine
    B. Is 50% ionised at physiological pH
    C. Produces cardiac depression at a lower concentration
        than at which it produces convulsions
    D. Has antimicrobial activity
    E. Has antifungal activity

Q 16. Ritodrine

    A. Produces bradycardia
    B. May cause pulmonary oedema
    C. Increases uterine contraction
    D. Increases peripheral vascular resistance
    E. Can cause hyperkalaemia

Q 17. Propofol

    A. Has anticonvulsant properties
    B. Is water soluble
    C. May cause pain on injection
    D. Is an imidazole
    E. Is 64% protein bound

Q 18. Ondansetron

    A. May be useful to treat post-operative nausea and
        vomiting
    B. Is an antagonist at muscarinic receptors for
        acetylcholine
    C. Should be given by slow intravenous infusion
    D. Has a peripheral site of action
    E. Antagonises apomorphine induced vomiting

Q 19. End products of arachidonic acid metabolism include

    A. Prostacyclin
    B. Bradykinin
    C. Leukotrienes
    D. Angiotensin
    E. Thromboxane

Q 20. Temazepam

A. Is available for parenteral injection
B. Is a GABA receptor agonist
C. Has a shorter terminal half-life than midazolam
D. Can be antagonised by flumazenil
E. Has active metabolites

Q 21. Isoflurane

A. Does not depress respiration
B. Does not sensitise the heart to catecholamines
C. Provides an easy inhalational induction
D. Undergoes 0.2% metabolism
E. Has a minimum alveolar concentration (MAC) value of 0.75

Q 22. The following are well absorbed from the gastro-intestinal tract

A. Loperamide
B. Morphine
C. Cromoglycate
D. Neomycin
E. Prednisolone

Q 23. Opioid drugs

A. Activate receptors found on ligand gated ion channels
B. Can produce analgesia by a peripheral mechanism
C. Produce most of their useful effects by actions at μ-receptors
D. Mimic the endogenous peptide substance P
E. Are as effective intrathecally as they are systemically

Q 24. Aminoglycoside antibiotics can cause

A. Optic atrophy
B. Dizziness
C. Ototoxicity
D. Potentiation of competitive neuromuscular blocking agents
E. Nephrotoxicity

Q 25. Suxamethonium

    A. Is metabolised principally by acetylcholinesterase
    B. Has an active metabolite
    C. Should be used with caution in patients using ecothiopate eye drops for the treatment of glaucoma
    D. Is recommended for patients with burns
    E. May cause myoglobinaemia

Q 26. Propranolol

    A. Increases plasma renin concentrations
    B. May be useful in the treatment of migraine
    C. Is the beta adrenoceptor antagonist of choice in an asthmatic patient
    D. May be useful in the treatment of essential tremor
    E. Has some anxiolytic activity

Q 27. Dopamine antagonists

    A. Are useful to treat travel sickness
    B. May induce extrapyramidal reactions
    C. Are more useful to treat the negative rather than the positive symptoms of schizophrenia
    D. Are used in neuroleptanalgesia
    E. May cause vasodilation

Q 28. The following drugs have a bioavailability of more than 50%

    A. Gentamicin
    B. Propanolol
    C. Morphine
    D. Atenolol
    E. Methadone

Q 29. The following drugs act via enzyme inhibition

    A. Allopurinol
    B. Physostigmine
    C. Indomethacin
    D. Meptazinol
    E. Enoximone

Q 30. The following drugs influence the rate of gastric emptying

  A. Morphine
  B. Ranitidine
  C. Metoclopramide
  D. Sucralfate
  E. Misoprostol

Q 31. Following drugs have clinically significant effect on opioid receptors

  A. Clonidine
  B. Pentazocine
  C. Diazepam
  D. Nalorphine
  E. Ketocyclazocine

Q 32. Drugs having agonist action at opioid receptors include

  A. Diacetyl morphine
  B. Naltrexone
  C. Naloxone
  D. Pentazocine
  E. Buprenorphine

Q 33. Enflurane

  A. Is a halogenated hydrocarbon
  B. Is more potent than halothane
  C. Has a boiling point within 5°C of that of halothane
  D. Potentiates competitive neuromuscular blockade
  E. Is metabolised to release fluoride

Q 34. Atropine

  A. Is an isomer of hyoscine
  B. May produce hyperpyrexia in children
  C. May increase anatomical dead space
  D. Is D-isomer of hyoscine
  E. Crosses the blood-brain barrier

Q 35. When given intravenously following produce mydriasis

- **A.** Phenylephrine
- **B.** Neostigmine
- **C.** Glycopyrrolate
- **D.** Pancuronium
- **E.** Trimetaphan

Q 36. Diazepam

- **A.** Has anticonvulsant properties
- **B.** Has an elimination half-life of less than 6 h
- **C.** Is metabolised to oxazepam
- **D.** Is soluble in water
- **E.** Has an imidazole ring in its structure

Q 37. Dantrolene sodium

- **A.** Has muscle relaxant property
- **B.** Is a respiratory stimulant
- **C.** Is useful in treating malignant hyperthermia
- **D.** Is an opiate antagonist
- **E.** A calcium channel blocker

Q 38. Atracurium

- **A.** Is degraded by Hoffmann elimination
- **B.** Is degraded by ester hydrolysis
- **C.** Is metabolised by glucuzonide transfer
- **D.** Is metabolised to one or more active metabolites
- **E.** Must be stored at 40°C

Q 39. The following readily cross blood-brain barrier

- **A.** Tubocurarine
- **B.** Atropine
- **C.** Lidocaine
- **D.** Neostigmine
- **E.** Physostigmine

Q 40. pH changes alter structure of

- **A.** Midazolam
- **B.** Atracurium

C. Suxamethonium
D. Thiopentone
E. Methohexitone

Q 41. Plasma cholinesterase activity may be reduced by

A. Malnutrition
B. Individuals heterozygous for the fluoride gene
C. An individual taking anticholinesterase eye drops
D. Ketamine
E. Stress

Q 42. The following drugs are recognised to cause diarrhoea

A. $MgSO_4$
B. Tetracycline
C. Glycopyrolate
D. Senna
E. Lactulose

Q 43. The following are natural precursors of epinephrine

A. Phenylalanine
B. Methionine
C. Dopamine
D. Norepinephrine
E. Isoprenaline

Q 44. Osmotic diuretics may cause

A. Hyponatraemia
B. Low plasma osmolality
C. Hypokalaemia
D. Increased blood volume
E. Raised intracranial pressure

Q 45. Thiazide diuretics

A. Act on the proximal convoluted tubule
B. Increase free water clearance
C. Increase calcium excretion
D. Increase uric acid excretion
E. Cause hyperglycaemia

Q 46. Ketamine may

    A. Increase the pulse rate
    B. Increase the blood pressure
    C. Cause muscle rigidity
    D. Cause delirium
    E. Reduce uterine tone

Q 47. Competitive neuromuscular blockade may be enhanced by

    A. Hypermagnesaemia
    B. Hypercalcaemia
    C. Lowering $PaCO_2$
    D. Lowering pH
    E. Aminoglycosides

Q 48. The following reduce systemic vascular resistance (SVR)

    A. Etomidate
    B. Enflurane
    C. Magnesium sulphate
    D. Ketamine
    E. Nitrous oxide

Q 49. Methaemoglobinaemia

    A. May be caused by higher oxides of nitrogen
    B. May be seen when prilocaine is used
    C. Is more likely to occur in myasthenic patients
    D. May be treated with methylene blue
    E. Is associated with lidocaine

Q 50. Class 1 calcium antagonists such as verapamil

    A. Can precipitate A-V block
    B. Increase afterload
    C. Reduce coronary vascular resistance
    D. Increase myocardial contractility
    E. Have more effect on heart muscle than peripheral blood vessel wall muscle

Q 51. Digoxin toxicity

- **A.** Is associated with ventricular bigemini
- **B.** May be alleviated by giving Ca^{2+}
- **C.** May be partly controlled by giving beta-blockers
- **D.** Is more likely to occur in hypokalaemia
- **E.** Is unlikely to occur at concentrations $<2\,ng/ml$

Q 52. The following have positive inotropic action

- **A.** Phenytoin
- **B.** Potassium
- **C.** Propranolol
- **D.** Glucagon
- **E.** Theophylline

Q 53. Isoprenaline

- **A.** Constricts blood vessels to skeletal muscle
- **B.** Causes bradycardia
- **C.** Is antagonised by propranolol
- **D.** Increases cardiac output
- **E.** May cause hyperglycaemia

Q 54. Lidocaine is used

- **A.** In VT post myocardial infarction
- **B.** In atrial extra systoles
- **C.** In ventricular extra systoles
- **D.** At a therapeutic concentration of $2-4\,\mu g/ml$
- **E.** To prolong the duration of phase 1 of the cardiac action potential

Q 55. Atropine

- **A.** Has an antidiuretic effect
- **B.** Can cause transient bradycardia
- **C.** Can increase intraocular pressure
- **D.** Relaxes ureteric muscle
- **E.** Has marked antimuscarinic and antinicotinic activity

Q 56. The following may cause bronchoconstriction

    A. Isoprenaline
    B. Atropine
    C. Theophilline
    D. Neostigmine
    E. Ritodrine

Q 57. The following are true of beta-blockers

    A. Efficacy is related to lipid solubility
    B. Metoprolol is relatively cardioselective
    C. Selectivity becomes less specific in higher doses
    D. Muscular fatigue is a common side effect
    E. Clinically useful drugs have no intrinsic beta agonist effect

Q 58. The nicotinic effect of acetylcholine is blocked by

    A. Atropine
    B. Curare
    C. Physostigmine
    D. Scopolamine
    E. Ergotamine

Q 59. Sodium nitroprusside (SNP)

    A. Is a vasodilator of arteries
    B. Is a vasodilator of veins
    C. Reduces myocardial contractility
    D. Shows marked tachyphylaxis
    E. Is metabolised via cyanide to form thiosulphate

Q 60. Nifedipine

    A. Is a Ca^{2+} channel blocker in cardiac and smooth muscle fibres
    B. Is well absorbed by mouth
    C. Undergoes less first-pass metabolism than verapamil
    D. Reduces SVR
    E. Is particularly useful in Woolf Parkinson White

Q 61. Atropine

    A. Is an isomer of hyoscine
    B. Increases physiological dead space

C. Causes methaemoglobinaemia

D. Can cause an increase in temperature

E. In low doses may decrease heart rate

Q 62. The following smooth muscle relaxants act by affecting calcium release

A. Dantrolene

B. Metolazone

C. Nifedipine

D. Verapamil

E. Prazosin

Q 63. Halothane

A. SVP at 20°C is about 1/3 of an atmosphere

B. Molecular weight is 196.4

C. Boiling point is 50.2°C

D. Contains four fluoride atoms

E. Can be used in an isoflurane vapouriser

Q 64. Isoflurane

A. Is a methyl ethyl ether

B. Increases A-V nodal conduction

C. Is a coronary vasodilator

D. Antagonises the effects of nifedipine

E. Does not increase cerebral blood flow

Q 65. Heparin

A. Should not be mixed with acidic solutions

B. Prolongs the clotting time but not the bleeding time

C. Inhibits thrombin

D. Can be reversed with vitamin K

E. Has a half-life of 30 min at therapeutic doses

Q 66. Ketamine induced hallucinations and delirium

A. Can be decreased by a benzodiazepine premed

B. Are less common in children

C. Are less common after short surgical procedures

D. Are less following i.m. administration

E. Are caused only by its metabolites

Q 67. Prilocaine

A. Is 70% protein bound

B. Is an amide

C. Is used in eutectic mixtures

D. Is metabolised by liver cholinesterase

E. Is more toxic than lidocaine at the same dose

Q 68. Ephedrine

A. Causes increased noradrenaline release from nerve terminals

B. Has bronchoconstrictor activity

C. Increases systemic vascular resistance

D. Reduces uterine tone

E. Displays tachyphylaxis

Q 69. The following decrease uterine muscle tone

A. Anti-diuretic hormone (ADH)

B. Salbutamol

C. Halothane

D. PGF2-alpha

E. Amyl nitrite

Q 70. Sulphonylureas

A. Increase peripheral utilisation of glucose

B. Are effective in patients with no endogenous insulin

C. Are used in type 2 diabetes mellitus

D. Can cause lactic acidosis

E. Do not cause hypoglycaemia

Q 71. Dextrans

A. Can interfere with blood clotting

B. Can cause renal failure

C. Can cause anaphylaxis

D. Decrease platelet aggregation

E. Are always presented in 5% dextrose

Q 72. Droperidol

   A. May cause hypoprolactinaemia
   B. Causes alpha-1-blockade
   C. Can cause parkinsonism
   D. Can cause a catatonic state
   E. Acts only on peripheral dopamine receptors

Q 73. Cimetidine

   A. Decreases lower oesophageal sphincter pressure
   B. Causes microsomal enzyme inhibition
   C. Is useful in treating acute anaphylaxis
   D. Decreases hepatic blood flow
   E. Inhibits gastric acid secretion

Q 74. Midazolam

   A. Is less potent than diazepam
   B. Has a half-life of 2 to 4 h
   C. Is 95% plasma protein bound
   D. Causes retrograde amnesia
   E. Reduces cerebral blood flow

Q 75. Bioavailability can be influenced by

   A. First pass metabolism
   B. Gastric acidity
   C. Plasma protein binding
   D. Gastrointestinal mucosa metabolism
   E. Renal clearance

Q 76. Thiazide diuretics may cause

   A. Hypokalaemic alkalosis
   B. Hyperuricaemia
   C. Increased blood glucose
   D. Hypercholesterolaemia
   E. Hyponatraemia

Q 77. The following cause raised intracranial pressure

   A. Ketamine
   B. Hypercapnia

C. Thiopentone
D. Halothane
E. Etomidate

Q 78. Aminoglycosides may cause

A. Optic atrophy
B. Tinnitus
C. Renal failure
D. Myasthenic syndrome
E. Hypothyroidism

Q 79. Ketamine

A. Is effective if given intrathecally
B. Stimulates respiration
C. Increases salivation
D. May be given orally
E. The R-isomer is a more potent analgesic than the S-isomer

Q 80. Halothane is associated with

A. Potentiation of the action of D-tubocurarine
B. A fall in body temperature
C. Decreased renal blood flow
D. Increased serum bromide levels
E. Trifluoroacetic acid in the urine

Q 81. Diazepam

A. Is water soluble
B. Is less potent in the elderly
C. Oral bioavailability is >80%
D. Has more than one active metabolite
E. Is an anticonvulsant

Q 82. Drugs used in the treatment of paroxysmal supraventricular tachycardia include

A. Verapamil
B. Nifedipine
C. Mexilitine

D. Lidocaine

E. Propranolol

Q 83. An hereditary enzyme abnormality may lead to altered metabolism of

A. Propofol

B. Aminophylline

C. Thiopentone

D. Suxamethonium

E. Atracurium

Q 84. Suxamethonium may cause

A. Bradycardia

B. Histamine release

C. Raised intraocular pressure

D. Salivation

E. Muscle pains

Q 85. Atracurium

A. Is degraded by ester hydrolysis

B. Is metabolised to laudanosine

C. In high doses acts faster than suxamethonium

D. Is potentiated by alkalosis

E. Is potentiated by alpha-adrenergic antagonists

Q 86. Nitrous oxide

A. Is stored as a liquid at room temperature

B. Is manufactured by heating ammonium nitrate

C. May be contaminated by nitric oxide

D. Reduces cerebral blood flow

E. In continuous use the pressure in a cylinder only falls when nearly empty

Q 87. Bupivacaine

A. Is a local anaesthetic of the amide group

B. Is metabolised by plasma cholinesterase

C. Can cause methaemoglobinaemia

D. Has a recommended maximum dose of 2 mg/kg
E. Can be used for post-operative pain relief

Q 88. The following local anaesthetic agents cause significant vasoconstriction

A. Cocaine
B. Amethocaine
C. Bupivacaine
D. Lidocaine
E. Prilocaine

Q 89. Halothane

A. Is an halogenated ether
B. Has a boiling point of 50°C
C. Delays cardiac conduction
D. Is metabolised to bromide ions
E. Is suitable for gaseous induction

Q 90. Isoflurane

A. Is a respiratory depressant
B. Is an halogenated ether
C. Has a MAC value of 0.76
D. Is metabolised less than halothane
E. Is a vasodilator

Q 91. Thiopentone sodium

A. Is an oxybarbiturate
B. Dilates cerebral vessels
C. Is acidic in solution
D. Is used as a 5% solution
E. May cause hypotension

Q 92. Nitrous oxide

A. In the UK is stored in cylinders at 4,400 kPa
B. Has a boiling point of 89°C
C. May cause agranulocytosis

D. Is eliminated by the lungs

E. Has a critical temperature of 36.5°F

Q 93. Atropine

A. Crosses the blood-brain barrier

B. Increases dead space

C. Is a bronchoconstrictor

D. Causes pyrexia

E. May cause bradycardia

Q 94. The following drugs are isomeric

A. Halothane

B. Enflurane

C. Isoflurane

D. Methohexitone

E. Thiopentone

Q 95. Insulin

A. Increases gluconeogenesis

B. Increases glycogen production

C. Stimulates the conversion of amino acids to protein in the liver

D. Raises intracellular potassium concentration

E. Is catabolic

Q 96. Etomidate

A. Lowers intraocular pressure

B. Is excreted in the urine

C. Causes pituitary suppression

D. Causes pain on injection

E. Is formulated in propylene glycol

Q 97. Compared with halothane, enflurane has

A. A higher boiling point

B. A lower SVP

C. A lower MAC

D. A higher molecular weight

E. A lower blood/gas solubility coefficient

Q 98. Alfentanil

A. Is reversed by naloxone

B. Has a shorter half-life than fentanyl

C. Is predominantly metabolised by the liver

D. Has a larger volume of distribution than fentanyl

E. May cause chest wall rigidity

Q 99. Oxygen

A. Is stored in cylinders at 137 kPa when full

B. Is stored in black cylinders

C. Has a critical temperature of 118°C

D. Is liquid in the cylinder

E. Supports combustion

Q 100. Carbon dioxide

A. Is stored in gaseous form

B. Is stored in green cylinders

C. Is stored at a pressure of 200 atm

D. Supports combustion

E. Has a critical temperature of 31°C

Q 101. Chlorpromazine

A. Is an alpha-blocker

B. Is a beta-blocker

C. May induce hypothermia

D. Is a butyrophenone

E. May cause sedation

Q 102. Compared to alfentanil, fentanyl has

A. A larger volume of distribution

B. A shorter half-life

C. Greater hepatic clearance

D. Higher pKa

E. Slower onset of action

Q 103. Oil/gas solubility of a volatile agent is related to

A. Potency
B. Speed of onset
C. Compatibility with soda lime
D. Arrhythmogenicity
E. Boiling point

Q 104. Flumazenil

A. Will reverse the sedative effects of diazepam
B. Can precipitate convulsions
C. Will reverse the sedative effects of fentanyl
D. Will reverse the sedative effects of halothane
E. Can cause ventricular arrhythmias

Q 105. The following values are correct for isoflurane

A. Boiling point = 60°C
B. MAC = 1.5 vol%
C. SVP = 243 mmHg
D. Blood/gas solubility coefficient = 1.4
E. Molecular weight = 185 daltons

Q 106. Gelatin solutions

A. Are not antigenic
B. Interfere with cross-matching
C. Have molecular weights averaging 100,000 dalton
D. May be urea linked
E. Remain in the circulation longer than dextrans

Q 107. Oxytocin

A. Acts only on the uterus
B. May cause water intoxication
C. Is secreted by the anterior lobe of the pituitary gland
D. Is active orally
E. Relaxes vascular smooth muscle

Q 108. Heparin

A. Carries an electropositive charge
B. Is a sulphated polypeptide

C. Is present with histamine in the mast cell
D. Affects thrombin
E. Has a half-life of 50 min after injection

Q 109. With regard to dantrolene sodium

A. Central effects are rare
B. Hepatotoxicity is a risk
C. Smooth and skeletal muscle are equally affected
D. It may be given orally
E. The action of the drug is to encourage the release of calcium ions from the sarcoplasmic reticulum

Q 110. Methohexitone

A. Is excreted mainly unchanged in the urine
B. Has four isomers
C. Is a thiobarbiturate
D. May cause pain on injection
E. Has a pH of 11

Q 111. Dantrolene

A. Has been used as a respiratory stimulant
B. Is only used in the treatment of malignant hyperpyrexia
C. Antagonises non-depolarising block
D. Relaxes skeletal muscle
E. Is supplied mixed with mannitol in ampoules

Q 112. Atropine

A. Causes contraction of GIT smooth muscle
B. Crosses the blood-brain barrier
C. Is a selective M-1 receptor antagonist
D. Increases dead space
E. Has antiemetic properties

Q 113. The following are side effects of metoclopramide

A. Migraine
B. Oculogyric crisis
C. Nausea

D. Increased prolactin secretion

E. Methaemoglobinaemia

Q 114. Frusemide may cause

A. Hypokalaemia

B. Hypoglycaemia

C. Raised serum urate

D. Increased renal blood flow

E. Deafness

Q 115. Lidocaine

A. Is a vasodilator

B. Is metabolised in the liver

C. Is an amide

D. Has a pKa of 7

E. Is a weak base

Q 116. An ideal intravenous induction agent

A. Will be stable in solution

B. Will be water soluble

C. Will have a high oil:water solubility coefficient

D. Crosses the placenta

E. Has a pKa of 11

Q 117. Hartmann's solution

A. Contains potassium ions

B. Equilibrates with extracellular fluid

C. Has a pH of 8

D. Is miscible with insulin

E. Contains no phosphate

Q 118. Halothane

A. Increases rate of gastric emptying

B. Increases cerebral blood flow

C. Is metabolised 20%

D. Has a MAC of 1.3

E. Is excreted renally

Q 119. **Lithium carbonate**

    A. Is used to treat manic-depressive psychosis

    B. Has to be administered by injection

    C. Has a rapid onset/offset of action

    D. Has a small therapeutic window

    E. Can cause diabetes insipidus

Q 120. **The following drugs are resistant to penicillinase**

    A. Phenoxymethylpenicillin

    B. Ampicillin

    C. Flucloxacillin

    D. Benzylpenicillin

    E. Methicillin

Q 121. **Vecuronium**

    A. Is a monoquaternary compound

    B. Has a shorter duration than pancuronium

    C. Is stable in water

    D. Is a benzyl isoquinolinium ester

    E. Crosses the placenta

Q 122. **Warfarin**

    A. Has little clinical effect for 36 h after a single dose

    B. May be reversed by protamine

    C. Is highly protein bound

    D. Is effective in vitro

    E. Interferes with the action of vitamin K

Q 123. **Spironolactone**

    A. Is a synthetic steroid derivative

    B. Acts on the proximal convoluted tubule

    C. Has antiandrogenic effects

    D. Reduces potassium and uric acid secretion

    E. Increases renal blood flow

Q 124. **The following cross the placenta membrane**

    A. Vecuronium

    B. Enflurane

C. Suxamethonium

D. Methohexitone

E. Alfentanil

Q 125. 2,6 Di-isopropylphenol

A. Has little protein binding in the plasma

B. Is more potent than thiopentone

C. Undergoes rapid renal metabolism

D. Is significantly excreted unchanged by the kidney

E. Releases histamine

Q 126. Propofol

A. Is a pale straw coloured liquid at room temperature

B. Is a free radical scavenger

C. Is formulated in soybean oil

D. Anaesthesia is normally maintained at blood levels of 0.5–1 mcg/kg

E. Has a molecular weight of 178 dalton

Q 127. First order kinetics

A. Are the most common kinetics encountered in drug metabolism

B. Multiple doses result in a steady state when first order kinetics apply

C. Can only occur in a single compartment model

D. Show the saturation phenomenon

E. Are represented by alcohol

Q 128. Non-competitive antagonists

A. Move the log dose-response curve for a drug to the right in a non-parallel manner

B. Reduce the gradient of the log dose-response curve

C. Have a response unrelated to their plasma concentration

D. Prevent a maximum agonal response

E. Display surmountability

Q 129. Non-steroidal anti-inflammatory drugs (NSAIDs)

A. Should not be used in hypertensive patients

B. Reduce platelet stickiness

C. Increase the effect of warfarin
D. Are available in parenteral form
E. Affect prostaglandin synthesis

Q 130. Tetracycline

A. Is active against Gram-positive and Gram-negative organisms
B. Causes necrotising enterocolitis
C. Does not cross the blood-brain barrier
D. Can enter bone
E. Should not be taken during pregnancy

Q 131. Naloxone

A. Produces dysphoria
B. Is >90% absorbed but has an oral bioavailability of <5%
C. Reverses pentazocine
D. Can causes a rise in blood pressure
E. Is an H_2 agonist

Q 132. Flecainide

A. Is indicated in supraventricular arrhythmias
B. Markedly increases QRS duration
C. May be given orally
D. Is a negative inotrope
E. As a bolus, the dose is 20–30 mg/kg

Q 133. With regard to antiarrhythmic agents

A. Class I drugs block sodium channels
B. Class III drugs prolong the refractory period of the myocardium
C. Lidocaine belongs to class I
D. Beta-blockers belong to more than one group
E. Class I drugs have a wide variety of clinical applications

Q 134. Etomidate

A. Is a carboxylated imidazole
B. Has an ester link in its structure

C. Has a pH of 8.1
D. Causes muscle movements which are associated with epileptic-form changes on the EEG
E. Is approximately 75% protein bound

Q 135. In clinical trials

A. A trial can be set up without a hypothesis
B. Any trial should attempt to answer as many questions as possible
C. Randomisation between two groups is not essential
D. In a single blind study the subject does not know if an active agent or placebo is being administered
E. In a single blind study the investigator does not know if an active agent or placebo is being administered

Q 136. Alfentanil

A. Has a shorter duration of action then fentanyl
B. Is metabolised to norafentanil
C. Is less potent than fentanyl
D. Has a pKa of 7.4
E. Has a short half-life due to a low volume of distribution

Q 137. The blood/gas partition coefficient for an inhalational agent

A. Is described in kPa at 37°C
B. Defines the potency of an agent
C. Is related to the potency: the lower the partition coefficient, the greater is the potency
D. Is 12 for halothane
E. Is 0.47 for nitrous oxide

Q 138. The following are correct oil:gas partition coefficients

A. Nitrous oxide = 1.4
B. Halothane = 422
C. Enflurane = 98.5
D. Isoflurane = 168
E. Desflurane = 19

Q 139. The following are the recommended maximum doses for local anaesthetic drugs

A. Lidocaine = 7 mg/kg
B. Bupivacaine = 2 mg/kg
C. Prilocaine = 6 mg/kg
D. Bupivacaine with adrenaline = 4 mg/kg
E. Levobupivacaine = 3 mg/kg

Q 140. Nitrous oxide

A. Is below its critical temperature at room temperature
B. Will support combustion
C. Is involved in the Fink effect
D. Does not increase intracranial pressure in the presence of space occupying lesions
E. Was discovered by Humphrey Davy

Q 141. MAC

A. Varies with age
B. Is more than 100% for nitrous oxide
C. Is measured with 30% oxygen in nitrous oxide as the carrier gas mixture
D. Indicates the concentration necessary for induction of anaesthesia
E. Is an ED95 for the drug in question

Q 142. Anaesthetic vapours have the following values for MAC

A. Halothane – 0.7%
B. Enflurane – 1.6%
C. Isoflurane – 1.8%
D. Desflurane – 6%
E. Sevoflurane – 2.4%

Q 143. The following drugs are extensively metabolised in the liver

A. Nifedipine
B. Enalapril

C. Ketamine

D. Ditiazem

E. Etomidate

Q 144. With regard to pharmacokinetics

A. Plasma clearance is independent of the concentration of drug

B. The volume of distribution may be greater than the total body water

C. Protein binding in the plasma may reduce the volume of distribution

D. The plasma half-life gives an indication of the duration of action

E. In the doses usually employed, thiopentone has zero-order kinetics

Q 145. Solutions of hydroxyethyl starch (hetastarch, pentastarch)

A. Have a similar average molecular weight to albumin

B. Does not prolong the PT or APTT

C. Are eliminated via the kidney

D. Are taken-up into the reticuloendothelial system

E. Cause an increase in plasma volume more than the infused volume

Q 146. Bupivacaine

A. Is an amide local anaesthetic

B. Increases the speed of cardiac conduction

C. May be used in 0.25% solution for intravenous regional anaesthesia (IVRA)

D. The hyperbaric solution for spinal anaesthesia contains 60 mg/ml of dextrose

E. The 0.5% solution contains bupivacaine at a concentration of 50 mg/ml

Q 147. Etomidate

A. Is soluble in water

B. Potentiates non-depolarising muscle relaxants

C. Increases systemic vascular resistance

D. Increases cerebral blood flow

E. Can be used safely in patients with porphyria

Q 148. The metabolism of atracurium

A. Is predominantly (>90%) by Hoffmann elimination

B. Is inhibited by hypothermia

C. Is inhibited by increasing blood pH

D. Produces a metabolite with muscle relaxant activity

E. Produces a metabolite with vagolytic activity

Q 149. Class 1 anti-arrhythmic drugs

A. May prolong the intracellular action potential

B. May shorten the intracellular action potential

C. May have no effect upon the intracellular action potential

D. Include the beta-blockers

E. Potentiate fast sodium current

Q 150. The chemoreceptor trigger zone is affected by

A. Chlorpromazine

B. Haloperidol

C. Apomorphine

D. Tetrahydrocannabinol

E. Domperidone

Section 2 – Answers

A 1.   **A.** false   **B.** true   **C.** true   **D.** false   **E.** true

All instruments will possess damping which affects their dynamic response. This includes mechanical, hydraulic, pneumatic and electrical devices. Damping is an important factor in the design of any system. In a measurement system it can lead to inaccuracy of the readings or display. Underdamping can result in oscillation and overestimation of the measurement. Overdamping can result in underestimation of the measurement. Critical damping is a compromise resulting in the fastest steady state reading for a particular system, with no overshoot or oscillation.

Pinnock CA, Lin ES, Smith T. *Fundamentals of Anaesthesia*, 2nd Edn. Greenwich Medical Media Ltd, 2003, Section 4: Chapter 2

A 2.   **A.** false   **B.** true   **C.** false   **D.** false   **E.** false

Boyle's law states that in an ideal gas at a constant temperature, the pressure of a gas is inversely proportional to its volume. Charles' law states that in an ideal gas when temperature is measured on the absolute scale, the temperature of a gas kept at constant pressure is directly proportional to its absolute temperature. The gas laws can be applied to any gas.

Pinnock CA, Lin ES, Smith T. *Fundamentals of Anaesthesia*, 2nd Edn. Greenwich Medical Media Ltd, 2003, Section 4: Chapter 1

A 3.   **A.** false   **B.** true   **C.** false   **D.** false   **E.** false

The critical temperature of a gas is that temperature above which it cannot be liquefied by compression alone. Sublimation is the change of state from vapour to solid.

Pinnock CA, Lin ES, Smith T. *Fundamentals of Anaesthesia*, 2nd Edn. Greenwich Medical Media Ltd, 2003, Section 4: Chapter 1

A 4.   **A.** false   **B.** true   **C.** true   **D.** false   **E.** true

Correct SI units are:
- Length = metre (m)
- Power = watt (W)
- Frequency = hertz (Hz)
- Mass = kilogram (kg)
- Energy = joule (J)

Pinnock CA, Lin ES, Smith T. *Fundamentals of Anaesthesia*, 2nd Edn. Greenwich Medical Media Ltd, 2003, Section 4: Chapter 1

A 5.   **A.** true   **B.** true   **C.** true   **D.** false   **E.** true

In normal 70 kg adults, the PEFR is around 550 l/min. It can be measured by any flow measuring device, such as the peak flow meter or a pneumotachograph. PEFR declines with age but may be improved to some extent by training.

Pinnock CA, Lin ES, Smith T. *Fundamentals of Anaesthesia*, 2nd Edn. Greenwich Medical Media Ltd, 2003, Section 1: Chapter 2

A 6.   **A.** false   **B.** true   **C.** false   **D.** true   **E.** false

The amount of gas dissolved in a liquid decreases as the temperature of the liquid rises. It is proportional to the pressure of gas in contact with the liquid but is uninfluenced by the presence of other dissolved gases (see Dalton's law).

According to Henry's law, the partial pressure exerted by a dissolved gas is proportional to the concentration of gas molecules in solution, irrespective of molecular weight. At equilibrium, the partial pressure of gas in contact with a liquid exerts the same tension as the dissolved amount.

Pinnock CA, Lin ES, Smith T. *Fundamentals of Anaesthesia*, 2nd Edn. Greenwich Medical Media Ltd, 2003, Section 4: Chapter 1

A 7.   **A.** false   **B.** false   **C.** true   **D.** false   **E.** false

Laminar flow of gas through a tube is determined by the Hagen-Poiseuille equation. Flow is therefore proportional to the pressure drop across the ends of the tube and the fourth power of the diameter, but inversely related to the length. Flow is inversely proportional to the viscosity (not its square). Density of a gas does not play a part in determining the rate of laminar flow through a tube.

Pinnock CA, Lin ES, Smith T. *Fundamentals of Anaesthesia*, 2nd Edn. Greenwich Medical Media Ltd, 2003, Section 4: Chapter 1

A 8.   **A.** true   **B.** false   **C.** true   **D.** true   **E.** false

A thermistor is an electrical device (fused oxides of heavy metals) which can be used in the measurement of temperature due to its change in resistance with temperature (non-linear decrease in resistance with increasing temperature) – hence the application in a Wheatstone bridge circuit. Thermistors are small and robust. Dissimilar junctional metals are thermocouples.

Pinnock CA, Lin ES, Smith T. *Fundamentals of Anaesthesia*, 2nd Edn. Greenwich Medical Media Ltd, 2003, Section 4: Chapter 2

A 9.   **A.** true   **B.** true   **C.** true   **D.** true   **E.** true

The SI system describes base and derived units. One pascal is the pressure that exerts a force of $1 N/m^2$ of surface area. Hertz are the number of cycles of periodic activity per second. The joule is the energy expended in moving a resistive force of 1 N over 1 m. One newton is the force required to accelerate a mass of 1 kg at $1 m/s^2$. One coulomb is the charge that passes a point in an electrical circuit if 1 A flows for 1 s.

Pinnock CA, Lin ES, Smith T. *Fundamentals of Anaesthesia*, 2nd Edn. Greenwich Medical Media Ltd, 2003, Section 4: Chapter 1

A 10.   **A.** false   **B.** true   **C.** false   **D.** true   **E.** false

This question requires application of Ohm's law:

$$V = IR$$

$$5 \times 2V \text{ batteries in series} = 10V$$

therefore

$$10 = \text{current} \times 1,000,000$$

which equates to 0.00001 A, which is the same as 0.01 mA.

Pinnock CA, Lin ES, Smith T. *Fundamentals of Anaesthesia*, 2nd Edn. Greenwich Medical Media Ltd, 2003, Section 4: Chapter 1

A 11. **A.** true **B.** true **C.** false **D.** true **E.** true

Below a certain temperature level (the critical temperature) any gas can be liquefied by the application of pressure. Above its critical temperature, the substance cannot exist as a liquid however much pressure is applied. At its critical temperature, a liquid will change spontaneously into vapour without heat being required. In other words, the latent heat of vapourisation is zero.

Pinnock CA, Lin ES, Smith T. *Fundamentals of Anaesthesia*, 2nd Edn. Greenwich Medical Media Ltd, 2003, Section 4: Chapter 1

A 12. **A.** true **B.** true **C.** true **D.** true **E.** false

There are various methods for measuring the concentration of vapours in a breathing system. These belong to the continuous analyser group which comprises mass spectrometry, infrared absorption, polarography, ultraviolet absorption, paramagnetism and thermal conductivity. Discrete analysers such as chromatography devices are not used in clinical anaesthesia.

Pinnock CA, Lin ES, Smith T. *Fundamentals of Anaesthesia*, 2nd Edn. Greenwich Medical Media Ltd, 2003, Section 4: Chapter 2

A 13. **A.** false **B.** false **C.** false **D.** true **E.** false

The Bourdon gauge is used to measure pipeline and cylinder pressure on anaesthetic machines, the measuring scale is kPa or bar. Flow is controlled by rotameters and reducing valves change high to low pressure. In some circumstances, the pressure drop across an orifice can be used to estimate flow but Bourdon-type gauges do not suit this purpose.

Pinnock CA, Lin ES, Smith T. *Fundamentals of Anaesthesia*, 2nd Edn. Greenwich Medical Media Ltd, 2003, Section 4: Chapter 2

A 14. **A.** true **B.** true **C.** true **D.** true **E.** false

At critical velocity (when Reynold's number is exceeded), laminar flow becomes turbulent. Turbulent flow is proportional to the radius squared, root of the pressure drop and the reciprocals of length and density. Viscosity is unrelated.

Pinnock CA, Lin ES, Smith T. *Fundamentals of Anaesthesia*, 2nd Edn. Greenwich Medical Media Ltd, 2003, Section 4: Chapter 1

A **15.** **A.** true   **B.** true   **C.** true   **D.** true   **E.** true

Latent heat of vapourisation is defined as the energy in J/kg necessary to change a liquid to a vapour without a change in temperature. This is the major source of heat loss from the respiratory tract (10–15% of total basal heat loss occurs from the trachea) and it is zero at critical temperature. Latent heat of vapourisation is less at higher temperatures because more molecules in the liquid will approach the energy level for leaving the vapour state.

Pinnock CA, Lin ES, Smith T. *Fundamentals of Anaesthesia*, 2nd Edn. Greenwich Medical Media Ltd, 2003, Section 4: Chapter 1

A **16.** **A.** true   **B.** true   **C.** true   **D.** false   **E.** false

A large plate area is necessary to avoid heating effects at the indifferent site. Good blood supply will also minimise this risk. A sinusoidal waveform is used for cutting and a damped sine wave for coagulation. Frequencies used vary between 300 kHz to 3 MHz and higher harmonics will exceed these values. Isolated circuits without earthing ('floating') avoid diathermy current leaking to earth.

Pinnock CA, Lin ES, Smith T. *Fundamentals of Anaesthesia*, 2nd Edn. Greenwich Medical Media Ltd, 2003, Section 4: Chapter 1

A **17.** **A.** false   **B.** true   **C.** true   **D.** false   **E.** true

The ideal size of water droplets for humidification is 5–10 microns. Smaller droplets will descend to the alveoli and larger ones will condense in the trachea. Scalding is a risk associated with water bath types when the temperature within exceeds 37°C. Colonisation of humidifiers with bacteria presents a potential infection risk. Nebulisers are more efficient than water bath types. The Bernoulli effect describes the drop in pressure occurring at a jet, where velocity is greatest, which is employed to draw up water from a reservoir. This effect is used in spinning disc and gas driven humidifiers among others.

Pinnock CA, Lin ES, Smith T. *Fundamentals of Anaesthesia*, 2nd Edn. Greenwich Medical Media Ltd, 2003, Section 4: Chapter 1

A 18. **A.** false **B.** true **C.** true **D.** false **E.** true

Boyle's law can be applied to any gas and states that PV = a constant, for a given temperature: therefore, as pressure increases, volume decreases.

Boyle's bottle is a glass vapourising device originally used for ether.

Pinnock CA, Lin ES, Smith T. *Fundamentals of Anaesthesia*, 2nd Edn. Greenwich Medical Media Ltd, 2003, Section 4: Chapter 1

A 19. **A.** false **B.** true **C.** true **D.** false **E.** true

Cooling is related to ambient temperature. The recommended environmental temperature is 22°C. Foil 'space-type' blankets reduce heat loss from radiation and warmed fluids and humidified inspired gases also reduce heat loss.

Phenothiazines exacerbate cooling because of their alpha blocking, vasodilating effect.

Pinnock CA, Lin ES, Smith T. *Fundamentals of Anaesthesia*, 2nd Edn. Greenwich Medical Media Ltd, 2003, Section 2: Chapter 11

A 20. **A.** false **B.** true **C.** true **D.** false **E.** true

One mole of a gas is a gram molecular weight, occupies 22.4 l at standard temperature and pressure (0°C and 101.3 kPa) and contains Avogadro's number of molecules. The volume is constant between gases at a given temperature. Above critical temperature, no gas can be liquefied by the application of pressure alone.

Pinnock CA, Lin ES, Smith T. *Fundamentals of Anaesthesia*, 2nd Edn. Greenwich Medical Media Ltd, 2003, Section 4: Chapter 1

A 21. **A.** true **B.** true **C.** false **D.** false **E.** true

Vapourisation of a liquid is facilitated by higher temperature. As a Bourdon gauge measures gas pressure, it can, although indirectly, measure a change in temperature as related to the pressure of gas within a container. The amount of gas that will dissolve in a liquid is primarily related to pressure. Increasing temperature will reduce the amount of gas that will dissolve. The oxyhaemoglobin dissociation curve moves to the right with a rise in temperature. SVP increases with temperature.

Pinnock CA, Lin ES, Smith T. *Fundamentals of Anaesthesia*, 2nd Edn. Greenwich Medical Media Ltd, 2003, Section 2: Chapter 8, Section 4: Chapter 1

A 22. **A.** true **B.** true **C.** false **D.** false **E.** true

The rate of diffusion of a gas through a membrane is directly related to the pressure gradient exerted, the membrane surface area and the diffusion coefficient for that gas. Diffusion is inversely related to thickness and molecular weight (slower diffusion through a thick membrane and with high molecular weight – Graham's law states that the rate of diffusion of a gas is inversely proportional to the square root of its molecular weight). High solubility confers rapid diffusion.

The diffusion coefficient is proportional to solubility divided by the square root of molecular weight.

Pinnock CA, Lin ES, Smith T. *Fundamentals of Anaesthesia*, 2nd Edn. Greenwich Medical Media Ltd, 2003, Section 2: Chapter 8, Section 4: Chapter 1

A 23. **A.** false **B.** false **C.** true **D.** true **E.** true

The Seebeck effect applies to themocouple. Thermistors have a non-linear relationship between resistance and temperature. Thermistors 'age' and their resistance changes with time. They exhibit hysteresis and have negative temperature coefficients.

Pinnock CA, Lin ES, Smith T. *Fundamentals of Anaesthesia*, 2nd Edn. Greenwich Medical Media Ltd, 2003, Section 4: Chapter 2

A 24. **A.** true **B.** false **C.** true **D.** false **E.** false

Pressure is defined as force per unit area. It is not concerned with flow. Manometer type devices such as a mercury column can be used to measure pressure. The SI unit of pressure is the pascal, which exerts a force of one newton per square metre.

Pinnock CA, Lin ES, Smith T. *Fundamentals of Anaesthesia*, 2nd Edn. Greenwich Medical Media Ltd, 2003, Section 4: Chapter 1

A **25.** **A.** false **B.** true **C.** false **D.** true **E.** true

SI units can be either fundamental or derived. The SI unit of temperature is kelvin. The candela is the SI unit of luminosity. Metre per second is a unit of velocity which is derived. Ampere is the SI unit of current. The mole is the SI unit of molecular numbers.

Pinnock CA, Lin ES, Smith T. *Fundamentals of Anaesthesia*, 2nd Edn. Greenwich Medical Media Ltd, 2003, Section 4: Chapter 1

A **26.** **A.** false **B.** false **C.** false **D.** true **E.** false

Light absorption of haemoglobin of both types is equal at the isobestic point of 805 nm. The presence of pigments such as carboxyhaemoglobin, methaemoglobin and bilirubin can cause inaccuracies in readings, although pigmentation of the skin does not modify the readings. The program within oximeter software 'searches' for a pulsatile signal thereby excluding venous flow.

Pinnock CA, Lin ES, Smith T. *Fundamentals of Anaesthesia*, 2nd Edn. Greenwich Medical Media Ltd, 2003, Section 4: Chapter 2

A **27.** **A.** false **B.** false **C.** true **D.** true **E.** false

Most surgical diathermy machines deliver power of 50 to 500 W at frequencies between 300 kHz and 3 MHz. Unipolar and bipolar diathermy are both used, bipolar is safer in patients with a cardiac pacemaker because unipolar systems may cause pacemaker inhibition. In unipolar diathermy, the indifferent electrode should provide a large surface area of good contact to avoid isolated areas of high current density which can cause burning.

Pinnock CA, Lin ES, Smith T. *Fundamentals of Anaesthesia*, 2nd Edn. Greenwich Medical Media Ltd, 2003, Section 4: Chapter 1

A **28.** **A.** false   **B.** false   **C.** false   **D.** false   **E.** true

Class 1 equipment is fully earthed. Class 2 equipment is double insulated. Class 3 is low voltage (<24 V). The patient should be isolated from electrical earth at all times. The specification of electrical equipment for use in wet areas and outside follows a different system (the IP system).

Pinnock CA, Lin ES, Smith T. *Fundamentals of Anaesthesia*, 2nd Edn. Greenwich Medical Media Ltd, 2003, Section 4: Chapter 1

A **29.** **A.** false   **B.** false   **C.** true   **D.** true   **E.** false

Absolute humidity is the mass of water vapour present in a given volume of gas at specified temperature and pressure. Relative humidity is the mass of water vapour in a given volume of gas as a percentage of the mass of water vapour required to saturate the gas at the same temperature and pressure. Ideally, relative humidity in the operating theatre should exceed 50% to reduce static electricity build-up. The electrical conductivity of some substances varies with water absorption and these types of electrical humidity transducers are used in most air-conditioning units. Regnault's hygrometer is based on the dew point of ether in a silvered tube and should not be confused with the hair hygrometer.

Pinnock CA, Lin ES, Smith T. *Fundamentals of Anaesthesia*, 2nd Edn. Greenwich Medical Media Ltd, 2003, Section 4: Chapter 2

A **30.** **A.** true   **B.** false   **C.** true   **D.** false   **E.** true

Doppler ultrasound uses an array of transducer crystals to transmit and receive ultrasound through a layer of silica gel which is necessary to prevent reflection. Doppler ultrasound uses the Doppler shift in frequency of the transmitted ultrasound waves to measure systolic and diastolic pressures. Signals are prone to movement artifact and are distorted by diathermy and arrhythmias.

Pinnock CA, Lin ES, Smith T. *Fundamentals of Anaesthesia*, 2nd Edn. Greenwich Medical Media Ltd, 2003, Section 4: Chapter 2

A **31.** **A.** true **B.** false **C.** true **D.** true **E.** false

Laminar flow is by definition smooth and occurs parallel to the walls of the cylinder. Laminar flow can only persist in straight, smooth-walled tubes without bends or constrictions. Outside these conditions Reynold's number is exceeded and turbulent flow results. For laminar flow, resistance is inversely proportional to the fourth power of the radius. For turbulent flow, flow is inversely proportional to the square root of the density.

Pinnock CA, Lin ES, Smith T. *Fundamentals of Anaesthesia*, 2nd Edn. Greenwich Medical Media Ltd, 2003, Section 4: Chapter 1

A **32.** **A.** false **B.** true **C.** false **D.** false **E.** false

EEG signals vary between 1–500 μV and 0–60 Hz. ECG signals vary between 0.1–50 mV and 0–100 Hz. EMG signals vary between 0.01–100 mV and 0–1,000 Hz (1 kHz). Signal-to-noise ratio is the ratio of signal amplitude to noise amplitude in decibels.

Pinnock CA, Lin ES, Smith T. *Fundamentals of Anaesthesia*, 2nd Edn. Greenwich Medical Media Ltd, 2003, Section 4: Chapter 2

A **33.** **A.** false **B.** false **C.** true **D.** true **E.** true

The rotameter is a constant flow, variable-orifice device. The Fleisch pneumotachograph has a set of tubes that are fixed and ensure laminar flow over a wide range. In a rotameter, when flow is mostly turbulent (i.e. at higher flows) gases of similar density will give approximately the same values. If the bobbin does not rotate freely, static may be keeping it in contact with the tube. In this situation, the orifice is disturbed and laminar flow is prevented, and thus the reading will not necessarily be accurate. At the narrowest part of a venturi, acceleration of flow causes a pressure drop, which is usually employed to cause entrainment.

Pinnock CA, Lin ES, Smith T. *Fundamentals of Anaesthesia*, 2nd Edn. Greenwich Medical Media Ltd, 2003, Section 4: Chapter 2

A **34.** **A.** false **B.** false **C.** false **D.** true **E.** true

Charles' law states that at constant pressure the volume of a mass of gas varies directly with the absolute temperature.

Boyle's law states that PV = a constant, thus pressure and volume are inversely related. At absolute zero, the theoretical volume of an ideal gas is zero. Real gases have liquefied before this point. Avogadro's hypothesis states that at a given temperature and pressure, 1 mole of any gas will occupy 22.4 l. Boyle's, Charles' and Gay-Lussac's law are combined to form the ideal gas law.

Pinnock CA, Lin ES, Smith T. *Fundamentals of Anaesthesia*, 2nd Edn. Greenwich Medical Media Ltd, 2003, Section 4: Chapter 1

A 35. **A.** false **B.** false **C.** false **D.** false **E.** true

The amount (or mass) of water present compared to the maximum amount possible at a given temperature is a definition of relative humidity. The mass of water in a unit volume of gas at a given temperature and pressure is absolute humidity. If droplets are present, supersaturation has occurred and relative humidity exceeds 100%. Relative humidity compares humidity present at the prevailing ambient pressure and temperature to that when fully saturated. Full saturation of inspired gas is possible.

Pinnock CA, Lin ES, Smith T. *Fundamentals of Anaesthesia*, 2nd Edn. Greenwich Medical Media Ltd, 2003, Section 4: Chapter 1

A 36. **A.** true **B.** false **C.** true **D.** true **E.** false

Air bubbles within the monitoring system decrease the resonant frequency and increase damping. Compliant tubing reduces accuracy due to wall movement, but rigid catheters will increase accuracy. Blood clots increase flow resistance and resonant frequency declines. A fixed zero point is necessary to avoid hydrostatic errors. Ideally, transducers will have a very high frequency response.

Pinnock CA, Lin ES, Smith T. *Fundamentals of Anaesthesia*, 2nd Edn. Greenwich Medical Media Ltd, 2003, Section 4: Chapter 2

A 37. **A.** true **B.** false **C.** false **D.** false **E.** true

The paramagnetic analyser relies on the paramagnetic properties of oxygen molecules and the readout is displayed as a percentage. Mass spectrometry can be used to measure all gases, but water vapour can interfere with sampling. Infrared absorption of light occurs where the gas or vapour contains molecules of two or more dissimilar atoms: it is not effective as a measuring device for oxygen although it can provide breath-by-breath analysis of vapours. In principle, the Haldane apparatus measures gas volumes on absorption of the gas, but there are problems in estimation of gases containing nitrous oxide. The polarographic or Clarke electrode consumes oxygen.

Pinnock CA, Lin ES, Smith T. *Fundamentals of Anaesthesia*, 2nd Edn. Greenwich Medical Media Ltd, 2003, Section 4: Chapter 2

A 38. A. true **B.** true **C.** true **D.** true **E.** true

The Rayleigh refractometer utilises the refractive index of a gas to calculate its concentration. Thermal conductivity is used in katharometers. In these devices, the cooling of a wire causes a change in resistance proportional to gas concentration. Solubility is employed in devices such as rubber strips when an increase in length accompanies gas absorption. Light emission features in the Raman light scattering measurement device. Both infrared and ultraviolet absorption are used in gas concentration measurement.

Pinnock CA, Lin ES, Smith T. *Fundamentals of Anaesthesia*, 2nd Edn. Greenwich Medical Media Ltd, 2003, Section 4: Chapter 2

A 39. A. false **B.** false **C.** true **D.** false **E.** true

A specific laser source emits light of a single frequency, the waves of which are in phase with minimal spread. The source is of low power (10 W or less). However, the concentration of the waves results in very effective heating at a single point. Class 1 lasers are the least dangerous (e.g. those found in a CD player). All surgical lasers fall into Class 4, as they are designed to burn or cut tissue and are therefore also a fire hazard.

Pinnock CA, Lin ES, Smith T. *Fundamentals of Anaesthesia*, 2nd Edn. Greenwich Medical Media Ltd, 2003, Section 4: Chapter 1

A 40. A. true **B.** true **C.** false **D.** false **E.** true

Pressure can be measured using a wire strain gauge, as stretching or compression of a wire will change its electrical resistance.

The inductance of a coil can be varied by changing the position of the magnetic core within, which may be related to the application of pressure. The optical defocussing manometer relies on the defocussing of a beam of light to alter the balance of light absorption between two photocells when the beam passes through a chamber in which a certain pressure is exerted. The change in pressure occurring at a narrowing describes the venturi principle. Although the pressure drop is proportional to flow, direct measurement of pressure is difficult. Torricellian vacuum exists above a column of mercury in a manometer: this is the principle of the common barometer for measuring atmospheric pressure.

Pinnock CA, Lin ES, Smith T. *Fundamentals of Anaesthesia*, 2nd Edn. Greenwich Medical Media Ltd, 2003, Section 4: Chapter 1

A 41. **A.** true **B.** false **C.** false **D.** true **E.** true

The Wheatstone bridge circuit is used to measure resistance by a principle of R1 + R2 = R3 + R4 and its sensitivity is only limited by the accuracy of the galvanometer. Small changes in resistance are usually detectable. An AC energised bridge can be used to measure very small changes in capacitance. The output from a bridge can be linearised if the signal is routed to an operational amplifier whose input resistance greatly exceeds those in the bridge circuit.

Pinnock CA, Lin ES, Smith T. *Fundamentals of Anaesthesia*, 2nd Edn. Greenwich Medical Media Ltd, 2003, Section 4: Chapter 1

A 42. **A.** false **B.** false **C.** false **D.** false **E.** true

Ohm's law applies to Ohmic conductors and can be stated as the current flowing through a conductor is directly proportional to the voltage, if the physical conditions (e.g. temperature) stay the same. The equation can be stated as $V = IR$. Ohm's law can be applied to direct or alternating current circuits. The filament of a light bulb changes temperature (and therefore resistance) with changes in the current, so the filament is not an Ohmic conductor. Resistors in series are additive and the voltage across each resistor is in proportion to the resistance.

Pinnock CA, Lin ES, Smith T. *Fundamentals of Anaesthesia*, 2nd Edn. Greenwich Medical Media Ltd, 2003, Section 4: Chapter 1

A 43. **A.** true   **B.** true   **C.** false   **D.** false   **E.** false

The metre is the basic unit of length and kelvin is the basic unit of temperature. Pascal is a derived unit of pressure, watt is the derived unit of power and coulomb is the derived unit of electrical charge.

Pinnock CA, Lin ES, Smith T. *Fundamentals of Anaesthesia*, 2nd Edn. Greenwich Medical Media Ltd, 2003, Section 4: Chapter 1

A 44. **A.** true   **B.** false   **C.** false   **D.** true   **E.** true

A SI unit of measurement of pressure is the pascal, one pascal being defined as the pressure that exerts a force of $1\,N/m^2$ of surface area. Pressure is a force and work will occur if the force moves through a distance. This adds another dimension to the units.

Pinnock CA, Lin ES, Smith T. *Fundamentals of Anaesthesia*, 2nd Edn. Greenwich Medical Media Ltd, 2003, Section 4: Chapter 1

A 45. **A.** true   **B.** true   **C.** false   **D.** false   **E.** false

In laminar flow, the fluid at the centre of the tube is flowing faster than at the sides, thus producing a conical profile. According to the Hagen-Poiseuille law, flow is proportional to the reciprocal of the fluid viscosity and the fourth power of the tube diameter. Inertial properties of the fluid (which depend on fluid density) are used to calculate Reynold's number, which determines the presence or absence of laminar flow. In the normal trachea during quiet breathing, turbulent flow will occur at peak flow rates.

Pinnock CA, Lin ES, Smith T. *Fundamentals of Anaesthesia*, 2nd Edn. Greenwich Medical Media Ltd, 2003, Section 4: Chapter 1

A 46. **A.** false   **B.** true   **C.** true   **D.** true   **E.** false

An inductor consists of coils of wire wrapped around a magnetisable core such as iron. It will act as a plain, low resistance to a constant current but the phases of voltage and current separate in alternating current circuits so that maximum current flows as the voltage passes through zero. The impedance of an inductor increases as the frequency of the alternating current increases.

Pinnock CA, Lin ES, Smith T. *Fundamentals of Anaesthesia*, 2nd Edn. Greenwich Medical Media Ltd, 2003, Section 4: Chapter 1

A 47. A. true **B.** false **C.** false **D.** false **E.** false

For conditions of laminar flow, Poiseuille's equation applies. Flow is therefore directly proportional to the pressure gradient across the cannula and the fourth power of its radius. Flow rate is inversely related to the viscosity of the fluid, which decreases with increasing temperature and length of the tube.

Pinnock CA, Lin ES, Smith T. *Fundamentals of Anaesthesia*, 2nd Edn. Greenwich Medical Media Ltd, 2003, Section 4: Chapter 1

A 48. A. true **B.** true **C.** true **D.** true **E.** true

The principle factor determining inertial properties of a fluid is the kinematic viscosity which is the ratio of viscosity to density. Note also that viscosity is dependent on temperature. Osmolality affects density of a liquid and surface tension acts as an inertial force which will oppose the commencement of flow.

Pinnock CA, Lin ES, Smith T. *Fundamentals of Anaesthesia*, 2nd Edn. Greenwich Medical Media Ltd, 2003, Section 4: Chapter 1

A 49. A. true **B.** true **C.** true **D.** false **E.** false

Surface tension is a force (measured in N/m) acting at the surface of a liquid due to attraction between liquid molecules. The law of Laplace relates surface tension to the radius of a bubble. If a spherical membrane is filled with fluid, the membrane wall will exert a force per unit length related to the wall thickness. Surface tension is related to temperature as temperature alters the viscosity of the liquid.

Pinnock CA, Lin ES, Smith T. *Fundamentals of Anaesthesia*, 2nd Edn. Greenwich Medical Media Ltd, 2003, Section 4: Chapter 1

Physics and Clinical Measurement

Answers

A 50. A. true **B.** false **C.** false **D.** false **E.** false

The cathode ray oscilloscope relies on a ramp voltage on the horizontal electrodes to create the horizontal deflection of the timebase. The electrode beam is a form of radiation that is deflected by an electrostatic charge on the plates and this radiation is converted to visible light by the fluorescence of the chemicals on the inner surface of the screen when struck by the beam. An electrostatic charge may also build up on the screen. When applied to the vertical deflection electrodes, a direct current will result in a movement of the baseline whereas an alternating current will result in the appearance of a waveform on the screen.

Parbrook GD, Davis PD, Kenny G. *Basic Physics and Measurement in Anaesthesia*. Butterworth-Heinemann, 1995

A 51. A. true **B.** true **C.** true **D.** true **E.** false

Viscosity of a fluid is its resistance to flow. Haemoglobin concentration, or haematocrit is the main influence on blood viscosity (exponential increase). Viscosity will change with plasma protein concentration. There is an increase with age. Blood viscosity changes with flow rates due to streaming of the cells in the middle of the vessel. There is no change with pressure unless pressure changes result in change in flow.

Yentis S, Hirsch N, Smith G. *Anaesthesia A to Z*. Butterworth-Heinemann, 1995

A 52. A. true **B.** true **C.** true **D.** true **E.** true

Viscosity is the tendency of a liquid or gas to resist flow. It can be measured in liquids using a viscometer, which measures the time that a liquid takes to travel through a fine bore tube. Also, liquid viscosity can be measured by placing the sample between two drums, turning the outer drum and measuring the torque on the inner drum (the dual drum technique). In a liquid, viscosity decreases as temperature increases and the converse is true for gases. The units of measurement are Ns/m^2 or the poise (named after Poiseuille).

Yentis S, Hirsch N, Smith G. *Anaesthesia A to Z*. Butterworth-Heinemann, 1995

A 53. **A.** false **B.** true **C.** false **D.** false **E.** true

Sound is measured using the SI unit of the decibel which is the ratio of two amounts of acoustic signal power equal to ten times the common logarithm of this ratio. It compares the power of the measured sound to that produced at the threshold of hearing. The normal range of hearing for humans is 20–20,000 Hz, the upper limit of which deteriorates with age. The average pain threshold is 130 decibels. Both sound and ultrasound can be focussed using acoustic lenses and mirrors.

A 54. **A.** false **B.** true **C.** true **D.** false **E.** true

The venturi effect describes the entrainment of a fluid through a side arm into a low pressure area which has been produced by a constriction in a tube. It should not be confused with the Coanda effect, which applies to fluid mechanic switching systems in ventilator design. Venturi devices are used for oxygen therapy, scavenging and suction equipment. A Bain circuit may be tested for integrity by the venturi test, whereby an inflated reservoir bag will empty if high gas flow is passed down the inner tube.

Pinnock CA, Lin ES, Smith T. *Fundamentals of Anaesthesia*, 2nd Edn. Greenwich Medical Media Ltd, 2003, Section 4: Chapter 1

A 55. **A.** true **B.** true **C.** true **D.** false **E.** true

The Coanda effect is similar to the venturi effect, in that gas accelerating through a nozzle (as a form of constriction) causes a pressure drop locally that may then be used to cause other actions. The effect is used in ventilator design to cause fluidic switching of jet streams. It is said that a similar flow alteration may occur beyond constrictions in blood vessels, for example atheromatous plaques in coronary arteries.

Pinnock CA, Lin ES, Smith T. *Fundamentals of Anaesthesia*, 2nd Edn. Greenwich Medical Media Ltd, 2003, Section 4: Chapter 1

A 56. **A.** true **B.** true **C.** false **D.** true **E.** false

The variable performance face mask has a plastic body with side holes on both sides. The holes allow venting of expired gas and entrainment of air. When there is no tidal flow from the patient, oxygen can accumulate in the mask so increasing the concentration and washing out carbon dioxide. The concentration of oxygen inspired by the patient is dependent on the oxygen flow and patient's respiratory pattern.

Pinnock CA, Lin ES, Smith T. *Fundamentals of Anaesthesia*, 2nd Edn. Greenwich Medical Media Ltd, 2003, Section 1: Chapter 1

A 57. A. false **B.** false **C.** true **D.** false **E.** true

The venturi mask (Ventimask) delivers a predetermined fixed concentration of oxygen at a flow higher than the patient's inspiratory flow rate. For example, a 24% oxygen valve requires an oxygen flow rate of 2 l/min and entrains air at a rate of 38 l/min. An increase in oxygen concentration requires a change of venturi valve and an increase in oxygen flow is required. The dead space is low and rebreathing does not occur because of the high flow of gas.

Pinnock CA, Lin ES, Smith T. *Fundamentals of Anaesthesia*, 2nd Edn. Greenwich Medical Media Ltd, 2003, Section 1: Chapter 4

A 58. A. true **B.** true **C.** true **D.** true **E.** true

A Fleisch or screen pneumotachograph uses the principle of pressure drop across a fixed resistance (orifice) to measure flow. The 'orifice' may consist of multiple narrow ducts (Fleisch) or a gauze screen but the flow must be laminar. Thermodilution measurement of cardiac output utilises the Fick principle. The Doppler effect is the change of frequency of reflected high frequency sound waves and is utilised to measure blood flow in vessels in vivo. The Wright's respirometer uses a spinning vane to measure gas flow. A bubble flowmeter is an historical alternative to the rotameter to measure gas flow on an anaesthetic machine.

Pinnock CA, Lin ES, Smith T. *Fundamentals of Anaesthesia*, 2nd Edn. Greenwich Medical Media Ltd, 2003, Section 4: Chapter 2

A 59. A. false **B.** false **C.** true **D.** true **E.** false

The electromagnetic flowmeter relies on the principle of Faraday's law of electromagnetic induction. It is a complete unit in a single probe that utilises an alternating current to generate the magnetic field and so provide more accurate results. The size of the probe is now sufficiently small to allow its use for intravascular measurement. The probe has to be either within the vessel or directly around the vessel: it cannot be used for transcutaneous measurements.

Pinnock CA, Lin ES, Smith T. *Fundamentals of Anaesthesia*, 2nd Edn. Greenwich Medical Media Ltd, 2003, Section 4: Chapter 2

A 60. **A.** false **B.** true **C.** true **D.** false **E.** false

The rotameter is a variable orifice flowmeter (an orifice has a diameter greater than its length). The tube is gas-specific, should be vertically mounted to avoid friction and the bobbin is scored so that it rotates to avoid sticking. The flow of the gas past the bobbin depends on the position of the bobbin: characteristically, laminar flow occurs close to the base and turbulent flow towards the top of the tube. The pressure drop across the bobbin will be dependent on the type of flow. The rotameter tube is calibrated for a specific gas at a specific pressure and temperature.

Pinnock CA, Lin ES, Smith T. *Fundamentals of Anaesthesia*, 2nd Edn. Greenwich Medical Media Ltd, 2003, Section 4: Chapter 2

A 61. **A.** false **B.** true **C.** true **D.** false **E.** false

Automated oscillometry machines over-read at low pressures and inflate to 20–30 mmHg above detected systolic pressure. These machines sense pulsations in the cuff; Korotkov sounds are heard by the operator in the manual occlusive cuff methods. Infrared plethysmography is utilised in the Penaz technique for digital pressure measurements. Doppler can be used to detect the change in arterial diameter pulsations during compression of the artery by an external cuff.

Pinnock CA, Lin ES, Smith T. *Fundamentals of Anaesthesia*, 2nd Edn. Greenwich Medical Media Ltd, 2003, Section 4: Chapter 2

A 62. **A.** false **B.** true **C.** false **D.** false **E.** false

Most capnographs in clinical use are based on the principle of infrared absorption. Normal end-tidal carbon dioxide is about

0.5–0.8 kPa less than arterial. Mainstream capnographs are quicker-reacting than sidestream types and use the head as sampling chamber, whereas sidestream types draw the sample into a small cuvette. The usual sampling rate for a sidestream capnograph is 50–500 ml/min.

Pinnock CA, Lin ES, Smith T. *Fundamentals of Anaesthesia*, 2nd Edn. Greenwich Medical Media Ltd, 2003, Section 4: Chapter 2

A **63.** **A.** true   **B.** false   **C.** false   **D.** true   **E.** true

Pneumotachographs are instruments used to measure flow. There are three main types: fixed resistance, hot wire and pitot. The most common instrument in use is the Fleisch or screen type, where flow is derived from a drop in pressure across a fixed resistance. Laminar flow is necessary to relate pressure drop to flow but although a low resistance is desirable, laminar flow is usually produced by having an arrangement of small-bore tubes or a mesh. The pressure gradient depends on gas composition including viscosity and temperature. All pneumotachographs can be used for breath-by-breath measurement.

Pinnock CA, Lin ES, Smith T. *Fundamentals of Anaesthesia*, 2nd Edn. Greenwich Medical Media Ltd, 2003, Section 4: Chapter 2

A **64.** **A.** true   **B.** true   **C.** false   **D.** false   **E.** true

Total body water can be estimated by indicator dilution techniques using antipyrine or deuterium oxide. Red cell mass is measured by using radioactive chromium labelled red cells. ECF volume is estimated by the use of radioactive sodium or chloride.

$$ICF = TBW - ECF$$

where ICF = intracellular fluid; TBW = total body water and ECF = extracellular fluid.

Plasma volume is measured by radioactive iodinated albumin.

Pinnock CA, Lin ES, Smith T. *Fundamentals of Anaesthesia*, 2nd Edn. Greenwich Medical Media Ltd, 2003, Section 2 : Chapter 2

A **65.** **A.** false   **B.** false   **C.** false   **D.** false   **E.** true

Extracellular fluid volume is about 14 l. Dilution techniques are used, but are not particularly accurate. Substances include sulphate, carbon labelled inulin and mannitol. Radiolabelled albumin is used to measure plasma volume and deuterium oxide is used to estimate total body water.

Pinnock CA, Lin ES, Smith T. *Fundamentals of Anaesthesia*, 2nd Edn. Greenwich Medical Media Ltd, 2003, Section 2: Chapter 2

A 66. **A.** false   **B.** false   **C.** true   **D.** true   **E.** true

Signal display may be analogue or digital. Digital methods include both LED and LCD types of display. Oscilloscopes, chart recorders and galvanometers are analogue. There are digital voltmeters available.

Pinnock CA, Lin ES, Smith T. *Fundamentals of Anaesthesia*, 2nd Edn. Greenwich Medical Media Ltd, 2003, Section 4: Chapter 2

A 67. **A.** false   **B.** true   **C.** true   **D.** true   **E.** true

The peak flow meter measures flow not volume. Wet spirometers (also known as Benedict-Roth type) are the most accurate method of measuring respiratory volumes. The vitalograph measures expired volume over time and can yield indices such as the FEV_1. A pneumotachograph measures gas flow but volume measurement is possible indirectly by integration of the flow signal over time.

Pinnock CA, Lin ES, Smith T. *Fundamentals of Anaesthesia*, 2nd Edn. Greenwich Medical Media Ltd, 2003, Section 4: Chapter 2

A 68. **A.** false   **B.** false   **C.** false   **D.** false   **E.** false

None of these devices can generate a flow-volume loop.

Pinnock CA, Lin ES, Smith T. *Fundamentals of Anaesthesia*, 2nd Edn. Greenwich Medical Media Ltd, 2003, Section 4: Chapter 2

A 69. **A.** false   **B.** false   **C.** false   **D.** false   **E.** false

Wright's respirometer is unaffected by the gas mixture. It may be placed at the catheter mount for convenience. The device will under-read if the vanes become wet and at low flow rates.

Pinnock CA, Lin ES, Smith T. *Fundamentals of Anaesthesia*, 2nd Edn. Greenwich Medical Media Ltd, 2003, Section 4: Chapter 2

A 70. A. true **B.** false **C.** true **D.** false **E.** true

HMEs can achieve about 60–70% relative humidity and warm gases to 29–34°C. Hot water bath humidifiers are prone to colonisation, particularly with pseudomonas. Droplets greater than 5 microns in diameter fall back into the container. Those of 2–4 microns tend to be deposited in the pharynx, while smaller droplets reach the bronchial tree.

Al-Shaikh B, Stacey S. *Essentials of Anaesthetic Equipment*, 2nd Edn. Churchill Livingstone, 2001

A 71. A. false **B.** true **C.** false **D.** false **E.** false

Boyle's law can simply be stated as PV = a constant.

It is therefore not specific to a given mass of gas. It applies to non-ideal gases. Pressure and temperature of a gas are described by Charles' law.

Pinnock CA, Lin ES, Smith T. *Fundamentals of Anaesthesia*, 2nd Edn. Greenwich Medical Media Ltd, 2003, Section 4: Chapter 2

A 72. A. true **B.** true **C.** true **D.** true **E.** true

One gram molecular weight of a gas contains Avogadro's number of molecules (6×10^{23}) and occupies 22.4 l at STP. It is equivalent to one mole.

Pinnock CA, Lin ES, Smith T. *Fundamentals of Anaesthesia*, 2nd Edn. Greenwich Medical Media Ltd, 2003, Section 4: Chapter 2

A 73. A. false **B.** false **C.** false **D.** false **E.** false

Critical temperature is the temperature above which a vapour cannot be compressed by the application of pressure alone. For oxygen the value is −118°C. The value for nitrous oxide is 36.5°C. Critical pressure is the pressure required to liquefy a vapour at its critical temperature.

Pinnock CA, Lin ES, Smith T. *Fundamentals of Anaesthesia*, 2nd Edn. Greenwich Medical Media Ltd, 2003, Section 4: Chapter 1

A 74. A. false **B.** false **C.** false **D.** true **E.** true

Critical pressure is the pressure required to liquefy a vapour at its critical temperature. The value for oxygen is 50 bar and for nitrous oxide 72 bar.

Yentis S, Hirsch N, Smith G. *Anaesthesia A to Z*. Butterworth-Heinemann, 1995

A 75. A. true **B.** true **C.** true **D.** false **E.** true

The cryoprobe is an instrument used to freeze tissue. Compressed gas (for example carbon dioxide or nitrous oxide) is passed through a narrowing. Expansion beyond this results in sudden gas expansion in which work is done and rapid cooling occurs (this is called the Joule-Thomson effect, an example of an adiabatic process). Cryoprobes work between −50 and −90°C.

Yentis S, Hirsch N, Smith G. *Anaesthesia A to Z*. Butterworth-Heinemann, 1995

A 76. A. true **B.** false **C.** false **D.** true **E.** true

An exponential decay process changes by constant proportion. The rate of decay is proportional to the amount of substance remaining at that time. The process will be 63% complete in one time constant, 87% in two and 95% complete in three time constants. The half-life is 69% of the time constant. The half-life of the process is constant.

A 77. A. true **B.** true **C.** false **D.** true **E.** false

Saturated vapour pressure (SVP) is the pressure exerted by the vapour phase of a substance above its liquid phase when the two are in equilibrium. At its boiling point, the SVP of a substance is equal to atmospheric pressure. SVP varies with both temperature and pressure, but relates to volatility rather than molecular weight *per se.*

Pinnock CA, Lin ES, Smith T. *Fundamentals of Anaesthesia*, 2nd Edn. Greenwich Medical Media Ltd, 2003, Section 4: Chapter 2

A 78. A. false **B.** true **C.** true **D.** true **E.** false

The working temperature inside a VIE is about $-160°C$. The critical temperature of oxygen is $-118°C$. Oxygen gas is evaporated and passes through the top of the tank. Liquid oxygen can be released via a control valve at the bottom of the tank if required. The VIE sits on a weighing scale to monitor the amount of liquid oxygen remaining.

Pinnock CA, Lin ES, Smith T. *Fundamentals of Anaesthesia*, 2nd Edn. Greenwich Medical Media Ltd, 2003, Section 4: Chapter 3

A 79. A. true **B.** true **C.** true **D.** false **E.** true

The curve on a volume vs pressure graph (called an isotherm) of nitrous oxide at a particular temperature above its critical temperature will follow a simple hyperbola reflecting the inverse relationship between pressure and volume for a gas (Boyle's law).

Pinnock CA, Lin ES, Smith T. *Fundamentals of Anaesthesia*, 2nd Edn. Greenwich Medical Media Ltd, 2003, Section 4: Chapter 1

A 80. A. false **B.** false **C.** true **D.** true **E.** false

The carbon dioxide electrode is included in most blood-gas analysers. A glass pH electrode and a silver/silver chloride reference electrode are incorporated and the system works on the principle of pH changes attributable to the formation of carbonic acid from carbon dioxide and water. The electrode is accurate and stable. The Clarke electrode measures oxygen and a lead anode is used in the galvanic fuel cell.

Pinnock CA, Lin ES, Smith T. *Fundamentals of Anaesthesia*, 2nd Edn. Greenwich Medical Media Ltd, 2003, Section 4: Chapter 2

A 81. A. true **B.** false **C.** false **D.** true **E.** false

Atmospheric air contains:
■ Oxygen – 21%
■ Nitrogen – 78%
■ Carbon dioxide – 0.03%

- Water vapour (to a variable degree)
- Inert gases are present at levels below 1%

Pinnock CA, Lin ES, Smith T. *Fundamentals of Anaesthesia*, 2nd Edn.
Greenwich Medical Media Ltd, 2003, Section 4: Chapter 1

A 82. A. true **B.** false **C.** false **D.** false **E.** false

Latent heat is the energy which is solely required to achieve a change of state without a change in temperature. It is greater at lower temperatures and less at high temperature. Specific latent heat is specified for a particular temperature. For example, the specific latent heat of vapourisation of water is 2.3 MJ/kg at 100°C.

Yentis S, Hirsch N, Smith G. *Anaesthesia A to Z*. Butterworth-Heinemann, 1995

A 83. A. false **B.** false **C.** true **D.** true **E.** true

The heat capacity of a body (C) is the amount of heat energy required to raise the temperature 1°C. It is obtained from the formula $C = Q/T$.

Specific heat capacity is the amount of heat energy required to raise the temperature of 1 kg of material by 1°C. The energy required to cause a change of state (without temperature change) is the latent heat.

Pinnock CA, Lin ES, Smith T. *Fundamentals of Anaesthesia*, 2nd Edn.
Greenwich Medical Media Ltd, 2003, Section 4: Chapter 1

A 84. A. true **B.** false **C.** false **D.** false **E.** false

The rate of diffusion of a gas across membranes is multifactorial and depends on molecular size, charge, solubility among others. Carbon dioxide is more soluble in blood than oxygen, is not charged, has no active transport and is a larger molecule than oxygen. The concentration gradient for oxygen is greater.

Pinnock CA, Lin ES, Smith T. *Fundamentals of Anaesthesia*, 2nd Edn.
Greenwich Medical Media Ltd, 2003, Section 2: Chapter 6

A 85. A. false **B.** true **C.** true **D.** true **E.** true

Diffusion obeys Graham's law. Nitrous oxide is less soluble than nitrogen in water. An increase in temperature will produce an increase in molecular movement and an increase in diffusion. Diffusion increases with an increase in membrane surface area. A higher pressure gradient results in a higher concentration gradient which leads to an increase in diffusion.

Pinnock CA, Lin ES, Smith T. *Fundamentals of Anaesthesia*, 2nd Edn. Greenwich Medical Media Ltd, 2003, Section 3: Chapter 1

A **86.** **A.** true **B.** true **C.** false **D.** true **E.** true

Fick's law states that the rate of diffusion across a membrane is proportional to the concentration gradient across the membrane. Graham's law states that the diffusion rate is inversely proportional to the square root of the density. As temperature rises, diffusion will increase. The thicker the membrane, the slower the rate of diffusion.

Pinnock CA, Lin ES, Smith T. *Fundamentals of Anaesthesia*, 2nd Edn. Greenwich Medical Media Ltd, 2003, Section 3: Chapter 1

A **87.** **A.** true **B.** false **C.** false **D.** false **E.** true

Osmolality is defined as the number of osmoles per kilogram of solvent. Osmolality of a solution can be estimated by measuring depression of the freezing point. Plasma osmolality is mainly due to sodium and its anions, normal plasma freezes at $-0.54°C$.

Pinnock CA, Lin ES, Smith T. *Fundamentals of Anaesthesia*, 2nd Edn. Greenwich Medical Media Ltd, 2003, Section 2: Chapter 2

A **88.** **A.** false **B.** true **C.** false **D.** true **E.** true

Osmolality is measured in osmoles/kg solvent (which is water in the body). Most of the contribution to the osmolality in plasma is due to sodium and its anions. Osmolality is slightly higher due to proteins and lipids. Depression of the freezing point can be used to measure the osmolality. The osmoreceptors in the hypothalamus regulate body fluid osmolality via anti-diuretic hormone.

Pinnock CA, Lin ES, Smith T. *Fundamentals of Anaesthesia*, 2nd Edn. Greenwich Medical Media Ltd, 2003, Section 2: Chapter 2

A 89. **A.** true   **B.** false   **C.** false   **D.** true   **E.** true

Absolute zero = −273.15°C

Triple point of water = 0.15°C

Kelvin (K) is the unit of the absolute temperature scale, one kelvin being 1/273.15 of the thermodynamic temperature of the triple point of water.

Alcohol boils at 78.5°C at standard atmospheric pressure and mercury freezes at −38.87°C.

Pinnock CA, Lin ES, Smith T. *Fundamentals of Anaesthesia*, 2nd Edn. Greenwich Medical Media Ltd, 2003, Section 4: Chapter 2

A 90. **A.** false   **B.** true   **C.** false   **D.** false   **E.** false

An increase in temperature results in an decreased viscosity of blood, an increased vapourisation of a volatile liquid, an increase in the voltage output from a thermocouple and a decrease in resistance of a thermistor. Carbon dioxide is less soluble with increasing temperature.

Pinnock CA, Lin ES, Smith T. *Fundamentals of Anaesthesia*, 2nd Edn. Greenwich Medical Media Ltd, 2003, Section 4: Chapter 2

A 91. **A.** true   **B.** true   **C.** true   **D.** true   **E.** true

The indifferent electrode is placed on the left shoulder.

Al-Shaikh B, Stacey S. *Essentials of Anaesthetic Equipment*, 2nd Edn. Churchill Livingstone, 2001

A 92. **A.** true   **B.** true   **C.** true   **D.** true   **E.** false

Heat loss can occur by movement of air away from exposed surfaces (convection): airflow currents such as laminar flow tents can increase heat loss further. Sweating from the skin can increase heat loss by a factor of ten and fluid loss can be as high as 2 l/h. Heat loss by infrared radiation from exposed portions of the body can be reduced by covering with a reflective 'space blanket'. As humidity increases, evaporation from the skin will decrease and so heat loss is reduced. The main site of heat loss from children is from the head as a child has a proportionally larger surface area of head to body than an adult.

Pinnock CA, Lin ES, Smith T. *Fundamentals of Anaesthesia*, 2nd Edn. Greenwich Medical Media Ltd, 2003, Section 2: Chapter 11

A **93.** **A.** false   **B.** true   **C.** false   **D.** true   **E.** false

Hypothermia is defined as a core temperature of less than 36°C. Evaporation from exposed tissue surfaces results in a rapid loss of heat and a rapid onset of hypothermia. Patients can be re-warmed both passively and actively and there must be adequate physiological and resuscitative support to control the hypotension, bradycardia and bradypnoea. As the body cools, shivering can occur which can increase the metabolic activity by up to 600% in adults.

Pinnock CA, Lin ES, Smith T. *Fundamentals of Anaesthesia*, 2nd Edn. Greenwich Medical Media Ltd, 2003, Section 2: Chapter 11

A **94.** **A.** false   **B.** true   **C.** false   **D.** true   **E.** true

The balloon on a pulmonary artery catheter is at the tip whereas the thermistor is 3.7 cm proximal to this. A small drop in accuracy occurs due to ageing but the accuracy is within 1°C. Pulmonary artery temperature equates to a core value. A thermistor consists of a small bead of semiconductor material. It has a negative temperature coefficient of resistance and a non-linear response.

Pinnock CA, Lin ES, Smith T. *Fundamentals of Anaesthesia*, 2nd Edn. Greenwich Medical Media Ltd, 2003, Section 4: Chapter 2

A **95.** **A.** true   **B.** true   **C.** false   **D.** false   **E.** false

A thermistor reacts more quickly than a thermocouple due to its small thermal capacity and may be used to measure flow, for example when incorporated into a pulmonary artery catheter. The response time is within 0.2 s. A thermistor is able to detect small temperature changes. The response is non-linear. The Seebeck effect relates to the thermocouple.

Pinnock CA, Lin ES, Smith T. *Fundamentals of Anaesthesia*, 2nd Edn. Greenwich Medical Media Ltd, 2003, Section 4: Chapter 2

A 96. **A.** false **B.** true **C.** false **D.** true **E.** false

Specific latent heat is the amount of energy needed to change the state of 1 kg of material at specified temperature. It is independent of mass and zero at critical temperature. Specific latent heat is greater at lower ambient temperatures.

Yentis S, Hirsch N, Smith G. *Anaesthesia A to Z*. Butterworth-Heinemann, 1995

A 97. **A.** false **B.** true **C.** false **D.** false **E.** false

The Wright respirometer is a spinning vane-type device usually termed an anemometer. Volume is obtained indirectly by integration of flow over time and the device can only measure volume up to 1,000 l. Humidity affects the accuracy of the device which is unidirectional.

Pinnock CA, Lin ES, Smith T. *Fundamentals of Anaesthesia*, 2nd Edn. Greenwich Medical Media Ltd, 2003, Section 4: Chapter 2

A 98. **A.** true **B.** true **C.** true **D.** true **E.** true

Humidity can be measured by the hair hygrometer, the dew point in Regnault's hygrometer and by direct weighing of water droplets after condensation. Humidity transducers measure a change in electrical conductivity of a material with humidity. The mass spectrometer can be used to measure the concentration of water vapour on a breath-by-breath basis.

Sykes K, Young D. *Respiratory Support in Intensive Care*. BMJ Books, 1999

A 99. **A.** false **B.** false **C.** false **D.** false **E.** true

Relative humidity is the mass of water vapour in a given volume of gas expressed as a percentage of the mass of water vapour required to saturate the same sample at identical temperature and pressure. Absolute humidity is the mass of water vapour present in a given volume of gas at defined temperature and pressure in grammes of water per cubic metre. Relative humidity increases with the passage of gas through the nose. The hair hygrometer will measure relative humidity over the range 15–85%. Relative humidity can be expressed as the ratio of actual water vapour pressure in a sample divided by saturated water vapour pressure.

Pinnock CA, Lin ES, Smith T. *Fundamentals of Anaesthesia*, 2nd Edn. Greenwich Medical Media Ltd, 2003, Section 4: Chapter 2

A 100. A. false **B.** true **C.** false **D.** false **E.** false

Modern diathermy machines are often electrically isolated, in which case they require no connection to the mains earth: the risk of shock is reduced by using floating patient circuits. Water will reduce the resistive path between two points especially if the water contains electrolytes. Dextrose solutions are safer for manometer lines. Electrolyte-containing solutions within manometer lines act as electrical conductors and thus suffer induced currents. Currents of a fraction of a milliampere at the myocardium are sufficient to cause ventricular fibrillation. A current as low as 150 μA contacting the heart via an intracardiac catheter may induce ventricular fibrillation.

Pinnock CA, Lin ES, Smith T. *Fundamentals of Anaesthesia*, 2nd Edn. Greenwich Medical Media Ltd, 2003, Section 4: Chapter 1

A 101. A. false **B.** false **C.** true **D.** true **E.** true

The patient and operating table are safer if they are independent of the mains electrical earth. Currents of a fraction of a milliampere are sufficient to cause ventricular fibrillation. Earthed mains equipment will always have a leakage current to earth which should be minimised in medical equipment. Wet hands will have a lower skin resistance than dry hands.

Pinnock CA, Lin ES, Smith T. *Fundamentals of Anaesthesia*, 2nd Edn. Greenwich Medical Media Ltd, 2003, Section 4: Chapter 1

A 102. A. false **B.** false **C.** false **D.** false **E.** true

A conducting floor, conducting shoes and a humid atmosphere are all features of an operating theatre that reduce the risk of static electricity to avoid explosions and fires when using flammable agents. They are all features that increase the risk of electrical shock, especially to staff. In both unipolar and bipolar diathermy, the patient is isolated from the electrical mains to reduce the risk of electrocution. The patient should be isolated from the mains earth to reduce the risk of a mains electrical shock.

Pinnock CA, Lin ES, Smith T. *Fundamentals of Anaesthesia*, 2nd Edn. Greenwich Medical Media Ltd, 2003, Section 4: Chapter 1

A 103. A. true   **B.** true   **C.** false   **D.** false   **E.** false

Diathermy requires high frequency current to generate its heating effect. The basic physical principle involved is that of current density. Provided that the indifferent electrode and active point are different in surface area, the same current flowing through each will generate a heating effect at the smaller due to its higher current density. Diathermy machines are usually not earthed. A complete circuit is necessary for current to flow.

Pinnock CA, Lin ES, Smith T. *Fundamentals of Anaesthesia*, 2nd Edn. Greenwich Medical Media Ltd, 2003, Section 4: Chapter 2

A 104. A. false   **B.** true   **C.** false   **D.** true   **E.** false

ECG measures potential difference between points, having a voltage range of 0.1–50 mV and a frequency range of 0–100 Hz. EMG signals vary between 0.01 and 100 mV with a frequency range of 0–1,000 Hz. EEG signals vary between 1 and 500 μV with a frequency range of 0–60 Hz.

Pinnock CA, Lin ES, Smith T. *Fundamentals of Anaesthesia*, 2nd Edn. Greenwich Medical Media Ltd, 2003, Section 4: Chapter 2

A 105. A. false   **B.** false   **C.** true   **D.** false   **E.** true

The Kelvin scale is a scale of temperature measurement which extends from absolute zero at −273° to boiling point of water at +373°. The scale defines the triple point of water as 273.16°. The Celsius scale varies from −273 which is absolute zero, to 100 which is the boiling point of water. Celsius was a Swedish scientist, Lord Kelvin (William Thomson) an Irish physicist.

Yentis S, Hirsch N, Smith G. *Anaesthesia A to Z*. Butterworth-Heinemann, 1995

A 106. A. false **B.** false **C.** true **D.** false **E.** false

Transducers convert one form of energy to another.
A transducer like a strain gauge, for example, converts
mechanical energy to electrical energy. Photoelectric cells are
transducers, converting light energy to electrical energy.
Amplifiers, transistors and oscilloscopes are not transducers.

Pinnock CA, Lin ES, Smith T. *Fundamentals of Anaesthesia*, 2nd Edn.
Greenwich Medical Media Ltd, 2003, Section 4: Chapter 1

A 107. A. false **B.** true **C.** true **D.** true **E.** false

A transducer converts one form of energy into another type.
Microphones, strain gauges and thermocouples are all
transducers. Oscilloscopes simply receive and display electrical
signals and the sphygmomanometer is a measurement device.

Pinnock CA, Lin ES, Smith T. *Fundamentals of Anaesthesia*, 2nd Edn.
Greenwich Medical Media Ltd, 2003, Section 4: Chapter 2

A 108. A. false **B.** false **C.** false **D.** true **E.** true

A strain gauge measures force, which can therefore
indirectly be related to pressure and mass (where mass is
acted on by gravity with a resultant force). An optical strain
gauge has been used for intravascular pressure measurement
(*Note:* not flow).

Sykes K, Young D. *Respiratory Support in Intensive Care.* BMJ Books, 1999

A 109. A. true **B.** false **C.** true **D.** true **E.** true

Amplifiers may be based on valves or semiconductors.
They do not change energy from one form to another, unlike
a transducer. The response of an amplifier is not necessarily
linear and the amplitude of noise and signal is increased.
Most biological signals require amplification before recording
due to their low signal strength.

Pinnock CA, Lin ES, Smith T. *Fundamentals of Anaesthesia*, 2nd Edn.
Greenwich Medical Media Ltd, 2003, Section 4: Chapter 2

A **110.** **A.** true **B.** false **C.** true **D.** true **E.** false

The beam is deflected in the x-axis by the time base, which is basically a saw tooth potential. Calibration of a CRO when used for ECG is 1 cm for 1 mV. The memory or storage oscilloscope is a digital variant which stores chunks of data digitally for later recall. The cathode ray tube may be polychromatic.

Parbrook GD, Davis PD, Kenny G. *Basic Physics and Measurement in Anaesthesia*. Butterworth-Heinemann, 1995

Pinnock CA, Lin ES, Smith T. *Fundamentals of Anaesthesia*, 2nd Edn. Greenwich Medical Media Ltd, 2003, Section 4: Chapter 2

A **111.** **A.** false **B.** true **C.** true **D.** true **E.** false

Ideally, the output of a nerve stimulator is a square wave, however factors within the circuit cause a 'rounding off' of the corners of the square wave. The optimal pulse length is 0.2 ms with a current amplitude of 0.5 to 5.0 mA for needle electrodes (nerve location) and a current amplitude of 10 to 40 mA for skin electrodes (neuromuscular blockade assessment). A tetanic stimulus can be between 50 Hz and 100 Hz. Train-of-four (TOF) uses 2 Hz stimulus for 0.2 ms. Skin electrodes suffer from skin resistance, implanted electrodes bypass skin resistance although resistance is only part of the formula – capacitance and inductance also play a part.

Pinnock CA, Lin ES, Smith T. *Fundamentals of Anaesthesia*, 2nd Edn. Greenwich Medical Media Ltd, 2003, Section 4: Chapter 2

A **112.** **A.** false **B.** true **C.** false **D.** true **E.** true

Optimal damping is 0.64 of critical damping and is a compromise producing the fastest response without excessive oscillations. Accuracy depends on as high a natural frequency of the system as possible. It should be 8–10 times the fundamental frequency (the maximum heart rate) and preferably over 100 Hz. This requires a non-compliant cannula, stiff transducer and the stiffest, narrow bore short tubing as is practical to push the system's mechanical resonances above the desired frequency response range of 0.5–40 Hz. Inevitably, the result is a compromise between speed of response and accuracy.

Pinnock CA, Lin ES, Smith T. *Fundamentals of Anaesthesia*, 2nd Edn. Greenwich Medical Media Ltd, 2003, Section 4: Chapter 2

A 113. A. true **B.** false **C.** true **D.** true **E.** false

An air bubble can be compressed and so will cause overdamping of the trace. If the taps are large bore, there is no change to the trace but a failed flushing system allows blood clots to form at the catheter, resulting in a damped trace. Elastic tubing results in an increase in damping. Silicone transducers are used in many of the disposable transducers in clinical practice: they are designed to reduce damping.

Pinnock CA, Lin ES, Smith T. *Fundamentals of Anaesthesia*, 2nd Edn. Greenwich Medical Media Ltd, 2003, Section 4: Chapter 2

A 114. A. false **B.** true **C.** false **D.** false **E.** false

An adult sphygmomanometer cuff width should be 14 cm wide or its width should be 20% greater than the diameter of the arm. Obesity leads to a cuff which is relatively too small leading to overestimation. Slow deflation will not affect accuracy. Positioning the mercury manometer above the arm will introduce zero error and result in underestimation. In atrial fibrillation the beat-to-beat variation in cardiac output resulting from the degree of atrial filling usually results in underestimation.

Pinnock CA, Lin ES, Smith T. *Fundamentals of Anaesthesia*, 2nd Edn. Greenwich Medical Media Ltd, 2003, Section 4: Chapter 2

A 115. A. false **B.** true **C.** false **D.** false **E.** true

The Penaz technique is a continuous, non-invasive method of measuring blood pressure. An infrared plethysmograph is mounted in a pneumatic cuff which is servo-controlled. Results are inaccurate in the presence of peripheral vascular disease and after 20 min or so it may become uncomfortable.

Pinnock CA, Lin ES, Smith T. *Fundamentals of Anaesthesia*, 2nd Edn. Greenwich Medical Media Ltd, 2003, Section 4: Chapter 2

A 116. A. false **B.** false **C.** true **D.** true **E.** false

Various patterns of stimulation are used in neuromuscular monitoring. The train-of-four describes four identical stimuli delivered at 2 Hz. Tetanic stimulation is used to detect fade at states of low receptor occupancy. Frequencies of 50 and 100 Hz are used. For single twitch stimulation a supramaximal stimulus is delivered at 1 Hz. Double burst stimulation was introduced to aid assessment of fade. Two tetanic bursts, each of three twitches at 20 ms intervals are used. The bursts are separated by 750 ms. For adequate respiration it is recommended that the T4/T1 ratio should exceed 70%.

Pinnock CA, Lin ES, Smith T. *Fundamentals of Anaesthesia*, 2nd Edn. Greenwich Medical Media Ltd, 2003, Section 4: Chapter 2

A 117. **A.** true   **B.** true   **C.** true   **D.** true   **E.** true

There are many methods available for the measurement of depth of anaesthesia. Evan's system is a clinical scoring system. Lower oesophageal contractility has been employed and in this instance both spontaneous and evoked contractions are recorded. Compressed spectral array uses the EEG power spectrum to produce a three-dimensional plot of cerebral activity. Evoked responses use auditory (AER) or visual (VER) stimuli to evoke brainstem (early) and early and late cortical responses. These responses may be attenuated or abolished by anaesthesia, sedation and sleep. Tunstall described the isolated forearm technique.

Pinnock CA, Lin ES, Smith T. *Fundamentals of Anaesthesia*, 2nd Edn. Greenwich Medical Media Ltd, 2003, Section 4: Chapter 2

A 118. **A.** true   **B.** true   **C.** true   **D.** false   **E.** true

The oximeter probe consists of two light emitting diodes (LED) that emit light at frequencies of 660 nm and 940 nm. Both shielding of the probe and sequential LED cycling minimise the effects of ambient light. Calibration of the oximeter is on volunteers down to a saturation of 80% with extrapolation below this level, therefore accuracy cannot be guaranteed below 80%. Some oximeters deliberately blank the display below 75%. There is a linear trend to underestimate the saturation as the concentration of haemoglobin falls; at haemoglobin levels of 8 g/100 ml, under-reading of up to 10–15% can occur. Carboxyhaemoglobin has a minimal absorption of 940 nm but has a similar absorbance to oxyhaemoglobin at 660 nm; this results in an overestimation of saturation.

Pinnock CA, Lin ES, Smith T. *Fundamentals of Anaesthesia*, 2nd Edn. Greenwich Medical Media Ltd, 2003, Section 4: Chapter 2

A 119. **A.** false **B.** true **C.** false **D.** true **E.** true

A distinction must be drawn between capnography, which is continuous measurement and graphic display of carbon dioxide concentration over time and capnometry, which is measurement only. Most common methods employ infrared spectroscopy although the mass spectrometer may also be used. The critical feature of capnographs is as short a response time as possible so as to be able to produce a continuous display. In COPD, the capnograph trace shows a steep upward slope due to expiratory obstruction but the plateau phase may slope and also be prolonged.

Yentis S, Hirsch N, Smith G. *Anaesthesia A to Z*. Butterworth-Heinemann, 1995

A 120. **A.** false **B.** true **C.** true **D.** false **E.** false

Most gases are repelled from a magnetic field and are called diamagnetic. Oxygen and nitric oxide are attracted to a magnetic field and are therefore termed paramagnetic. Paramagnetic molecules have two unpaired electrons spinning in the same direction in the outer electron shell. Paramagnetic analysers consist of a cell within a magnetic field suspended in which is a glass dumb-bell. The spheres of the dumb-bell are filled with nitrogen and the principle of measurement is the return of the system to a zero point after displacement. Paramagnetic analysers have a slow response time and cannot be used to measure nitrogen concentration as nitrogen is weakly diamagnetic.

Pinnock CA, Lin ES, Smith T. *Fundamentals of Anaesthesia*, 2nd Edn. Greenwich Medical Media Ltd, 2003, Section 4: Chapter 2

A **121.** **A.** true **B.** false **C.** true **D.** true **E.** true

The polarographic or Clarke electrode is used to measure blood oxygen tension although it can also be used to measure oxygen in a mixture of gases. It has a platinum cathode and a silver/silver chloride anode in a solution of electrolyte such as sodium or potassium chloride. It requires a voltage to drive it (unlike the fuel cell) and must be maintained at 37°C. Halothane is reduced by the voltage applied between the electrodes. This may cause falsely high readings. This will not occur if a membrane impermeable to halothane is used.

Pinnock CA, Lin ES, Smith T. *Fundamentals of Anaesthesia*, 2nd Edn. Greenwich Medical Media Ltd, 2003, Section 4: Chapter 2

A **122.** **A.** false **B.** true **C.** false **D.** true **E.** true

The Severinghaus carbon dioxide electrode is so named to avoid confusion with the oxygen electrode, usually named after Leland Clarke.

The carbon dioxide electrode consists of a glass pH electrode (in which the glass is permeable to hydrogen ions, thereby generating a potential depending on the pH difference between the inside and outside of the bulb electrode).

The bulb is covered with a film of electrolyte containing sodium bicarbonate and salt, and that film is covered by a membrane of teflon which is permeable to carbon dioxide gas but not to water or hydrogen ions. The carbon dioxide gas in a sample diffuses into the film and controls the pH of that electrolyte film, such that a ten-fold rise of pCO_2 lowers the pH of the electrolyte by 1.0 pH unit.

It is affected by temperature, so must be calibrated and used at a constant temperature, usually 37°C.

The glass is not permeable to carbon dioxide, and is (very slightly) permeable to H^+ ions. In order to measure the electrical potential created by a change of pH on the outside, very sensitive electronic amplification is needed, for example, the input resistance of the meter should be at least a million million Ohms.

Severinghaus JW, 2001 (personal communication)

A **123.** **A.** false   **B.** true   **C.** false   **D.** false   **E.** false

Rotameters are constant pressure drop – variable orifice devices. Flow is laminar at low levels, becoming turbulent at higher levels, but the glass tubes are calibrated to take this into account. It is important that the bobbin is able to spin freely and therefore the rotameters should stand upright. Static electricity will cause the bobbin to adhere to the side wall. Design features will reduce this liability. Modern rotameters will function accurately down to values of 200 ml/min.

Pinnock CA, Lin ES, Smith T. *Fundamentals of Anaesthesia*, 2nd Edn. Greenwich Medical Media Ltd, 2003, Section 4: Chapter 2

A **124.** **A.** false   **B.** false   **C.** true   **D.** true   **E.** true

Most capnographs in clinical use are based on infrared absorption. The response time of mainstream analysers is quicker than that of sidestream devices which require a pump to draw the sample (which is returned to the system) and a water trap to avoid water vapour contamination. Some inaccuracy is introduced into sidestream analysis by dead space gas in the sample tubing, but this may be minimised by good design.

Pinnock CA, Lin ES, Smith T. *Fundamentals of Anaesthesia*, 2nd Edn. Greenwich Medical Media Ltd, 2003, Section 4: Chapter 2

A **125.** **A.** true   **B.** false   **C.** true   **D.** true   **E.** true

Expiration of carbon dioxide is dependent on metabolic status and the integrity of the pulmonary circulation. In situations of increased metabolism (MH and exercise) end-tidal carbon dioxide rises. With falling cardiac output it will fall. When the pulmonary circulation becomes obstructed to a significant degree (pulmonary or air emboli for example) end-tidal carbon dioxide will fall.

Pinnock CA, Lin ES, Smith T. *Fundamentals of Anaesthesia*, 2nd Edn. Greenwich Medical Media Ltd, 2003, Section 4: Chapter 2

A **126.** **A.** false   **B.** false   **C.** false   **D.** true   **E.** false

The filling pressure in an oxygen cylinder is 137 bar (13,700 kPa), that of nitrous oxide 4,400 kPa. Oxygen exists in the cylinder as a vapour under pressure. Nitrous oxide is stored within the cylinder as a vapour in equilibrium with a liquid (until nearly empty, when vapour alone is present). Molybdenum is added to the steel for extra strength.

Pinnock CA, Lin ES, Smith T. *Fundamentals of Anaesthesia*, 2nd Edn. Greenwich Medical Media Ltd, 2003, Section 4: Chapter 2

A 127. **A.** false **B.** true **C.** true **D.** true **E.** false

Infrared light is absorbed by molecules composed of two or more dissimilar atoms, therefore water, nitrous oxide and halothane will interfere with the absorption of infrared light when used to measure carbon dioxide. Oxygen and helium will not absorb the infrared light.

Pinnock CA, Lin ES, Smith T. *Fundamentals of Anaesthesia*, 2nd Edn. Greenwich Medical Media Ltd, 2003, Section 4: Chapter 2

A 128. **A.** false **B.** false **C.** false **D.** true **E.** false

As temperature falls then measured oxygen tension will fall. There are nomograms available to estimate the changes. A pH electrode is used for direct measurement of pH. Standard bicarbonate is measured in a sample titrated to a pCO_2 of 5.3 kPa, this eliminates the respiratory component. The Clarke oxygen electrode described by Leland Clarke was the first oxygen electrode in which both cathode and anode were membrane covered to prevent protein deposition and therefore inaccuracy. Heparin being acid reduces the pH of the sample.

Pinnock CA, Lin ES, Smith T. *Fundamentals of Anaesthesia*, 2nd Edn. Greenwich Medical Media Ltd, 2003, Section 4: Chapter 2

A 129. **A.** false **B.** true **C.** false **D.** true **E.** true

Desflurane is highly volatile, having a boiling point of 23°C. In a vapouriser desflurane is heated to 39°C to raise its vapour pressure to 1,550 mmHg and this is mixed with fresh gas flow under pressure controlled conditions. This is an example of a measured flow vapouriser. In case of mains failure a battery backup is fitted to supply the heating element.

Pinnock CA, Lin ES, Smith T. *Fundamentals of Anaesthesia*, 2nd Edn. Greenwich Medical Media Ltd, 2003, Section 4: Chapter 3

A **130.** **A.** true **B.** true **C.** true **D.** false **E.** true

Gas chromatography is a contraction of the term gas-liquid chromatography. In this process one solvent is absorbed onto an inert material – the stationary phase, while a carrier gas (helium or nitrogen, for example) is passed over it. Temperature is usually programmed, starting constant and then increasing to a predetermined value. Various detection methods can be used including katharometers, flame ionisation and electron capture detection.

Sykes K, Young D. *Respiratory Support in Intensive Care*. BMJ Books, 1999

A **131.** **A.** true **B.** true **C.** true **D.** false **E.** false

In terms of gas measurement, methods may be specific or non-specific. Non-specific methods include: density, viscosity, thermal conductivity, refractive index and solubility. Specific methods include: paramagnetism, infrared absorption, ultraviolet absorption and mass spectrometry.

Sykes K, Young D. *Respiratory Support in Intensive Care*. BMJ Books, 1999

A **132.** **A.** true **B.** true **C.** false **D.** false **E.** true

Refractometers are capable of measuring the components of a gas mixture. They require calibration using known gas concentrations and are frequently used to calibrate vapourisers. The measurement is therefore indirect. Water vapour will affect the accuracy of refractometers.

Sykes K, Young D. *Respiratory Support in Intensive Care*. BMJ Books, 1999

A **133.** **A.** true **B.** true **C.** true **D.** true **E.** true

Raman scattering is similar to fluorescence. When gas molecules are bombarded with a discrete wavelength, the molecules scatter energy at a different wavelength, which can be measured. This system, although possible, is not in clinical use. Halothane absorbs infrared light at 3.3 μm, forming the basis of infrared absorption spectroscopy which is in common clinical use. Halothane also has a useful absorption bandwidth at 200 nm in the ultraviolet spectrum. This property is utilised in ultraviolet gas analysers. Mass spectrometers are the 'gold standard' for the measurement of complex gas mixtures, but online breath-by-breath analysis is fraught with difficulties. The Drager Narcotest is a simple device that utilises the change in tension in a silicone rubber strip on absorption of halothane. This device is relatively non-specific to vapours and has a slow response time. It is not in common clinical use.

Pinnock CA, Lin ES, Smith T. *Fundamentals of Anaesthesia*, 2nd Edn. Greenwich Medical Media Ltd, 2003, Section 4: Chapter 2

A **134. A.** false **B.** true **C.** false **D.** true **E.** false

The defibrillator contains a capacitor which is charged to 5,000 V designed to deliver a DC shock through an inductor which prolongs the exponential discharge characteristics. Some energy is lost in the inductor thus delivered energy is less than stored. Thoracic impedance is reduced by the first shock so successive shocks at the same set energy level deliver greater energy to the heart.

Pinnock CA, Lin ES, Smith T. *Fundamentals of Anaesthesia*, 2nd Edn. Greenwich Medical Media Ltd, 2003, Section 4: Chapter 2

A **135. A.** false **B.** true **C.** false **D.** false **E.** true

The Rubens valve is a non-rebreathing valve usually used in combination with self-inflating resuscitation bags. It has a bobbin and spring design which allows spontaneous breathing of room air in the expiratory position. The Rubens valve occasionally jams in the inspiratory position.

Davey AJ, Moyle JTB, Ward CS. *Ward's Anaesthetic Equipment*. WB Saunders, 1997

A 136. A. false **B.** true **C.** true **D.** false **E.** true

Entonox is a 50:50 mixture of oxygen and nitrous oxide which is stored in cylinders as a gas at 137 bar. The filling ratio is 0.75. It should be stored at room temperature to avoid separation.

Pinnock CA, Lin ES, Smith T. *Fundamentals of Anaesthesia*, 2nd Edn. Greenwich Medical Media Ltd, 2003, Section 1: Chapter 1

A 137. A. false **B.** false **C.** false **D.** true **E.** true

Entonox will separate and liquefy below −7°C (the so-called pseudocritical temperature). The cylinders are blue with blue/white shoulders. The mixture is stored as a gas at 13,700 kPa and should be kept vertical. The Poynting effect is the dissolution of oxygen into the nitrous oxide as it is bubbled through.

Pinnock CA, Lin ES, Smith T. *Fundamentals of Anaesthesia*, 2nd Edn. Greenwich Medical Media Ltd, 2003, Section 1: Chapter 1

A 138. A. false **B.** true **C.** false **D.** false **E.** false

Soda lime consists of a mixture of calcium (94%), sodium and potassium hydroxides. The mixture is supplied with about 20% water content and an indicator is added (usually turning from pink to white or white to violet when exhausted). The mixture should be tightly packed to avoid channelling. Soda lime is used for the deliberate absorption of carbon dioxide in circle systems.

Pinnock CA, Lin ES, Smith T. *Fundamentals of Anaesthesia*, 2nd Edn. Greenwich Medical Media Ltd, 2003, Section 1: Chapter 1

A 139. A. true **B.** false **C.** false **D.** false **E.** false

Helium is an inert gas present in the atmosphere. It is very poorly soluble and has a low density leading to its use when flow is turbulent (for example, upper airway obstruction). In lower airway obstruction, where the flow is predominantly laminar and therefore related to viscosity, helium and oxygen would have a higher viscosity than nitrogen and oxygen. This would theoretically make things worse. Helium is supplied in brown cylinders at 137 bar and is also available as heliox in a mixture with 21% oxygen.

Yentis S, Hirsch N, Smith G. *Anaesthesia A to Z*. Butterworth-Heinemann, 1995

A **140.** **A.** false   **B.** true   **C.** false   **D.** true   **E.** true

Nitrous oxide is an inhalational anaesthetic agent isolated first by Priestly in 1772. It has a critical temperature of 36.5°C (and is therefore a vapour rather than a gas at room temperature), a boiling point of −88°C and supports combustion. Side effects include marrow depression and spinal cord degeneration.

Pinnock CA, Lin ES, Smith T. *Fundamentals of Anaesthesia*, 2nd Edn. Greenwich Medical Media Ltd, 2003, Section 3: Chapter 5

A **141.** **A.** true   **B.** false   **C.** true   **D.** false   **E.** false

HAFOE stands for 'high air flow oxygen enriched' devices. The Bernoulli principle is used with a venturi device to cause entrainment of air around an oxygen jet venturi. These devices are constant in performance and require masks with holes to enable high volumes of air to be entrained.

Yentis S, Hirsch N, Smith G. *Anaesthesia A to Z*. Butterworth-Heinemann, 1995

A **142.** **A.** false   **B.** false   **C.** true   **D.** true   **E.** true

Medical gas cylinders are made of molybdenum steel (or aluminium) and are painted to a standard body/shoulder colour scheme. The gases/vapours should be free of water vapour which may freeze and block the outlet. They should not be stored near flammable materials such as oil or grease. Periodically the cylinder strength is tested by a hydraulic ram. The empty tare weight is stamped on the outside of each cylinder. A specific pin index system for attachment of the yoke prevents inadvertent errors in mounting.

Pinnock CA, Lin ES, Smith T. *Fundamentals of Anaesthesia*, 2nd Edn. Greenwich Medical Media Ltd, 2003, Section 1: Chapter 1

A **143.** **A.** true   **B.** false   **C.** true   **D.** false   **E.** false

Carbon dioxide is not supplied in pipeline form. Oxygen and nitrous oxide are supplied at 4 bar, as is entonox. Compressed air may be supplied at either 7 bar (for power tools) or 4 bar.

A **144.** **A.** true   **B.** true   **C.** false   **D.** true   **E.** false

Laser (light amplification by simulated emission of radiation) light is monochromatic and the photons are in phase. They are classified according to their degree of hazard. CD player lasers are Class 1 and safe whereas all surgical lasers are Class 4 as they are designed to damage tissue. The carbon dioxide laser is absorbed by water and therefore penetrates tissue poorly. It is used for superficial surgery. The argon laser, like the Nd-Yag laser, can be transmitted by optical fibres and can therefore be used endoscopically. Laser tubes are designed to withstand the effects of carbon dioxide and KTP laser beams. However, they will ultimately burn through and ignite like any other tube with prolonged exposure.

Pinnock CA, Lin ES, Smith T. *Fundamentals of Anaesthesia*, 2nd Edn. Greenwich Medical Media Ltd, 2003, Section 4: Chapter 1

A **145.** **A.** true   **B.** false   **C.** true   **D.** false   **E.** false

The Mapleson classification describes the characteristics of breathing systems. Mapleson A circuit is the Magill, also available as the Lack in coaxial format. The Mapleson D circuit is the Bain and the Jackson-Rees modification of Ayre's T piece (itself Mapleson E) is commonly used for paediatrics. The Mapleson A circuits are the most efficient for spontaneous respiration.

Pinnock CA, Lin ES, Smith T. *Fundamentals of Anaesthesia*, 2nd Edn. Greenwich Medical Media Ltd, 2003, Section 1: Chapter 1

A **146.** **A.** true   **B.** false   **C.** false   **D.** false   **E.** true

The Magill circuit is a Mapleson A circuit which is efficient for spontaneous respiration but not suitable for controlled respiration. In spontaneously breathing patients, alveolar minute volume alone (70 ml/kg/min) is sufficient to prevent rebreathing. The Magill circuit is not suitable for patients under 25 kg in weight. A coaxial version is available as the Lack circuit.

Pinnock CA, Lin ES, Smith T. *Fundamentals of Anaesthesia*, 2nd Edn. Greenwich Medical Media Ltd, 2003, Section 1: Chapter 1

A **147.** **A.** false **B.** true **C.** true **D.** true **E.** false

Time-cycled pressure generators generate relatively low pressure around 1.5 kPa. The flow pattern is that of a decreasing exponential function. The peak pressure will be related to airways resistance and changes in compliance (for example, reducing) reduces tidal volume. Small leaks will make little difference but, unlike flow generators, larger leaks result in under ventilation of the patient.

Yentis S, Hirsch N, Smith G. *Anaesthesia A to Z*. Butterworth-Heinemann, 1995

A **148.** **A.** false **B.** true **C.** false **D.** true **E.** false

The main constituent of soda lime is calcium hydroxide (94%). Sodium hydroxide (5%) is added to improve reactivity and for its hygroscopic properties. Potassium hydroxide (1%) is added to harden the granules and prevent powdering. The reaction is exothermic; the temperature inside a canister may reach 60°C. Water is added to enable the reaction to take place since carbon dioxide reacts with water to form carbonic acid which subsequently reacts with calcium hydroxide to form an end product of calcium carbonate.

Pinnock CA, Lin ES, Smith T. *Fundamentals of Anaesthesia*, 2nd Edn. Greenwich Medical Media Ltd, 2003, Section 1: Chapter 1

A **149.** **A.** false **B.** false **C.** true **D.** true **E.** true

The electroencephalogram is a varying voltage signal with amplitudes between 1 and 500 μV. The EEG is divided into 4 bands: alpha 8–13 Hz, beta >13 Hz, delta <4 Hz and theta 4–7 Hz. Deepening anaesthesia causes a progressive increase in signal amplitude with a reduced frequency.

Pinnock CA, Lin ES, Smith T. *Fundamentals of Anaesthesia*, 2nd Edn. Greenwich Medical Media Ltd, 2003, Section 4: Chapter 2

A **150.** **A.** false   **B.** false   **C.** false   **D.** false   **E.** true

For laminar flow, the Hagen-Poiseuille equation applies. Flow is directly related to the pressure gradient across the tube and the fourth power of the radius. Flow is inversely related to viscosity and length of the tube.

Pinnock CA, Lin ES, Smith T. *Fundamentals of Anaesthesia*, 2nd Edn. Greenwich Medical Media Ltd, 2003, Section 4: Chapter 2

A 1. **A.** true **B.** true **C.** false **D.** false **E.** false

Symptoms include headache, worse in the morning and on straining, nausea and vomiting. Signs include impaired conscious level, confusion, hypertension and bradycardia (Cushing's reflex), hypotension, apnoea and fixed dilated pupils. Rhinorrhoea is a sign of basal skull fracture.

Yentis S, Hirsch N, Smith G. *Anaesthesia A to Z*. Butterworth-Heinemann, 1995

A 2. **A.** true **B.** true **C.** true **D.** false **E.** false

The subclavian vein lies below and in front of the subclavian artery. The spinal cord ends at approximately L2 in adults. The subarachnoid space ends at S2 in adults.

A 3. **A.** true **B.** true **C.** true **D.** false **E.** true

Indications for surgical management include depressed skull fracture if depressed greater than skull thickness, most acute extradural and subdural haematomas, some intracranial mass lesions or haematomas, delayed hydrocephalus.

Gupta A, Summors A. *Notes in Neuroanaesthesia and Critical Care*. Greenwich Medical Media Ltd, 2001

A 4. **A.** true **B.** false **C.** true **D.** false **E.** true

Ventricular tachycardia with a palpable pulse would be an indication for synchronised DC cardioversion. In the case of pulseless VT, the VF protocol should be followed. Cardioversion in digoxin toxicity may precipitate severe arrhythmias and should be avoided.

A 5. **A.** false **B.** false **C.** true **D.** true **E.** false

The internal laryngeal nerve supplies the mucous membranes of the larynx above the vocal cords. The hypoglossal nerve is the motor nerve to the tongue muscles. The nucleus ambiguus is one of the three vagal nuclei. It is a motor nucleus found in the reticular formation of the medulla.

A 6. **A.** true **B.** true **C.** true **D.** false **E.** true

Dextrans reduce blood viscosity and reduce erythrocyte and platelet aggregation. Patients on the oral contraceptive pill and, more recently proven, hormone replacement therapy, are at increased risk.

A 7. **A.** true **B.** true **C.** true **D.** true **E.** false

Initially there is a shortened QT interval and narrow, peaked T waves. The QRS complex broadens and the p wave disappears. At plasma levels of 6–8 mmol/l VT and VF readily occur. At levels of 8–10 mmol/l the cardiac muscle fibres become unexcitable and the heart stops in ventricular diastole.

Pinnock CA, Lin ES, Smith T. *Fundamentals of Anaesthesia*, 2nd Edn. Greenwich Medical Media Ltd, 2003, Section 2: Chapter 5

A 8. **A.** false **B.** false **C.** false **D.** true **E.** false

Cycling into expiration occurs when airway pressure reaches the manually set level. Therefore, the cycling pressure is predetermined although the compliance will influence the rate at which it is reached and thus the inspiratory time and tidal volume.

A 9. **A.** true **B.** false **C.** true **D.** true **E.** false

The mode is the most frequently occurring observation. 68% of observations lie within ±1 SD and 99.7% lie within ±3 SD from the mean.

Standard deviation is a measure of the variability of the observations from the mean.

Swinscow TDV. *Statistics at Square One*. BMJ Group, 1980

A **10.** **A.** true **B.** false **C.** true **D.** true **E.** true

The standard error of the mean is the SD divided by the square root of the number of observations. It is a measure of the precision of an estimate of a population parameter.

Swinscow TDV. *Statistics at Square One*. BMJ Group, 1980

A **11.** **A.** true **B.** true **C.** true **D.** false **E.** true

Petechiae are found on the chest, upper limbs, axillae and conjunctiva. Fat globules may be found in the retina, urine or sputum.

Morgan GE, Mikhail MS. *Clinical Anaesthesiology*, 2nd Edn. Appleton and Lange, 1996

A **12.** **A.** true **B.** false **C.** false **D.** false **E.** false

The two other nerves in the '3 in 1' block are the obturator and lateral cutaneous nerve of the thigh. The femoral nerve lies lateral to the femoral artery and vein in its own fascial sheath.

Pinnock CA, Lin ES, Smith T. *Fundamentals of Anaesthesia*, 2nd Edn. Greenwich Medical Media Ltd, 2003, Section 1: Chapter 7

A **13.** **A.** true **B.** false **C.** false **D.** false **E.** true

Sustained head lift for 5 s suggests less than 30% blockade. Other indicators may be present at higher levels of blockade.

Pinnock CA, Lin ES, Smith T. *Fundamentals of Anaesthesia*, 2nd Edn. Greenwich Medical Media Ltd, 2003, Section 1: Chapter 4

A **14.** **A.** true **B.** true **C.** true **D.** false **E.** false

Other drugs used include lidocaine, diazepam, calcium and magnesium.

Yentis S, Hirsch N, Smith G. *Anaesthesia A to Z*. Butterworth-Heinemann, 1995

A **15.** **A.** true **B.** true **C.** false **D.** true **E.** true

Loss of CSF through the puncture site produces a low-pressure headache due to traction on the cranial meninges.

Pinnock CA, Lin ES, Smith T. *Fundamentals of Anaesthesia*, 2nd Edn. Greenwich Medical Media Ltd, 2003, Section 1: Chapter 7

A 16. A. false **B.** false **C.** true **D.** false **E.** false

The dose of adrenaline is 0.5–1.0 mg i.m. or 50–100 mcg i.v.

A 17. A. true **B.** false **C.** true **D.** true **E.** false

Mendelson's syndrome was originally described in 1946 in obstetric patients in which large airway obstruction occurred due to solid food particles.

Pinnock CA, Lin ES, Smith T. *Fundamentals of Anaesthesia*, 2nd Edn. Greenwich Medical Media Ltd, 2003, Section 1: Chapter 2

A 18. A. false **B.** true **C.** true **D.** true **E.** true

FRC is unchanged but closing capacity falls progressively with age.

Pinnock CA, Lin ES, Smith T. *Fundamentals of Anaesthesia*, 2nd Edn. Greenwich Medical Media Ltd, 2003, Section 2: Chapter 8

A 19. A. true **B.** true **C.** true **D.** false **E.** true

Risk factors for DVT may be classified according to the type of operation, patient factors and concomitant disease.

Surgical risk factors include duration of surgery greater than 30 min, major joint replacements, abdominal and pelvic surgery.

Patient factors include a previous history, thrombophilia, age >40, pregnancy, OCP, HRT, obesity, immobility, varicose veins (if having abdominal or pelvic surgery).

Concomitant diseases include recent MI, heart failure, malignancy, trauma, lower limb paralysis, haematological diseases, inflammatory bowel disease and nephrotic syndrome.

Allman K, Wilson I. *Oxford Handbook of Anaesthesia*. Oxford University Press, 2002

A 20. A. false **B.** false **C.** false **D.** true **E.** true

Although only patients who are ASA I or II would usually be considered suitable, some ASA III patients (for example chemotherapy patients) may be considered on an individual basis. Patients with significant heart or chest disease, insulin dependant diabetes or obesity are unsuitable. Surgery should not be expected to last for more than 1 h and should be relatively 'minor' in terms of risk of postoperative bleeding, pain and nausea. There must be adequate social support and adult supervision and the patient should live within one hour's travelling distance from the hospital. Alcohol and driving should be avoided for 24 h.

Allman K, Wilson I. *Oxford Handbook of Anaesthesia*. Oxford University Press, 2002

A 21. A. true **B.** true **C.** true **D.** true **E.** true

The rate of pneumothorax in the supraclavicular approach may be 1–6% and is more common in patients with chronic obstructive pulmonary disease (COPD). Horner's syndrome is caused by interruption of the sympathetic nerve supply to the head and is characterised by ipsilateral ptosis, meiosis, anhydrosis (lack of sweating) and nasal stuffiness. Convulsions are caused by intra-arterial injection and may occur with very small amounts of local anaesthetic. Other complications include haemothorax, recurrent laryngeal nerve block and extradural or spinal block. Bilateral blocks should not be performed.

Yentis S, Hirsch N, Smith G. *Anaesthesia A to Z*. Butterworth-Heinemann, 1995

A 22. A. true **B.** true **C.** false **D.** true **E.** true

The minimum alveolar concentration (MAC) is that which prevents movement to a standard skin incision in 50% of subjects studied.

MAC is increased in the very young, in chronic alcohol abuse and with hypernatraemia and acute sympathetic stimulation (such as by sympathomimetic drugs). MAC is decreased in the elderly, in hypo/hyperthermia, and with acute alcohol intoxication, severe anaemia, hypoxia and hypercarbia, MAP <40 mmHg, hypercalcaemia, hyponatraemia, pregnancy and multiple depressant drugs.

Since MAC is defined in terms of percentage of one atmosphere it is not altered by altitude.

Morgan GE, Mikhail MS. *Clinical Anaesthesiology*, 2nd Edn. Appleton and Lange, 1996

A 23. **A.** false **B.** false **C.** true **D.** true **E.** true

Scavenging systems work on low pressure and have built-in safety mechanisms such as pressure relief valves to prevent excessive positive or negative pressures. Scavenging may be active or passive. A passive system typically has a wide-bore copper pipe leading to the atmosphere outside. This may be affected by the wind or if mounted high up may result in back pressure due to the weight of denser anaesthetic vapours such as nitrous oxide.

Parbrook GD, Davis PD, Kenny G. *Basic Physics and Measurement in Anaesthesia*. Butterworth-Heinemann, 1995

Al-Shaikh B, Stacey S. *Essentials of Anaesthetic Equipment*, 2nd Edn. Churchill Livingstone, 2001

A 24. **A.** true **B.** true **C.** false **D.** true **E.** false

Chest compressions should be at a rate of 100/min and both single and multiple rescuer techniques should use a ratio of 15 compressions to 2 breaths. This is because coronary perfusion is higher and better maintained after 15 compressions than after 5 compressions. The recommended tidal volume is 700–1000 ml.

UK Resuscitation Guidelines, 2001

A 25. **A.** true **B.** false **C.** false **D.** true **E.** true

The coagulation cascade is activated by a disease process resulting in widespread fibrin clot formation, consumption of clotting factors (I, II, V and XIII) and platelets and secondary fibrinolysis. It may be associated with infection (especially gram-negative), placental abruption, amniotic fluid embolism, major trauma, burns, malignancy, hypoxia, hypovolaemia and severe liver disease. Laboratory investigations may reveal thrombocytopenia, prolonged INR, APTT and TT, normal or reduced fibrinogen, raised fibrin degradation products and d-dimers. Management is directed at the underlying cause and haemostatic support with platelets, fresh frozen plasma (FFP) and cryoprecipitate were appropriate. (Cryoprecipitate may be required if the fibrinogen level cannot be raised above 1 g/l by

FFP alone.) The use of heparin is controversial but may be indicated in patients with thromboembolic phenomena.

Pinnock CA, Lin ES, Smith T. *Fundamentals of Anaesthesia*, 2nd Edn. Greenwich Medical Media Ltd, 2003, Section 2: Chapter 3

A 26. A. true **B.** false **C.** false **D.** false **E.** true

Risk factors for air/gas embolism include spontaneous ventilation (due to the negative central venous pressure (CVP)), any open vein above the level of the heart, pressurised infusions, certain types of surgery (e.g. neurosurgery in the deck-chair position, orthopaedic (long bone), laparoscopic, vascular and ENT surgery). Symptoms and signs include severe chest pain, sudden fall in end-tidal carbon dioxide (ETCO$_2$), oxygen saturation, tachycardia, millwheel murmur (machinery murmur is heard in patent ductus arteriosus), sudden rise in CVP, asystolic cardiac arrest.

Management aims to prevent any further air/gas entering the circulation, limit the progress of an existing embolus and support the circulation. The surgeon should flood the wound with saline and compress major veins. Any open vein should be brought to a level below the heart. Nitrous oxide should be turned off and in laparoscopic surgery, the abdomen should be decompressed. Rapid IV fluids will increase CVP and placing the patient in the head down left lateral position is meant to keep any air or gas within the right atrium until it can be aspirated via a CVP line or until it dissolves.

Yentis S, Hirsch N, Smith G. *Anaesthesia A to Z*. Butterworth-Heinemann, 1995

Allman K, Wilson I. *Oxford Handbook of Anaesthesia*. Oxford University Press, 2002

A 27. A. false **B.** true **C.** false **D.** true **E.** false

Although rocuronium is used it does not strictly speaking represent a safe technique. If intubation fails the patient will not return to spontaneous ventilation before hypoxia ensues. In order to suppress the haemodynamic response to laryngoscopy and intubation, it may be necessary in at-risk patients to administer a short acting opioid prior to induction. This can be reversed with naloxone in the event of a failed intubation if required. Preoxygenation for 3–5 min with a close fitting face mask or 4–5 vital capacity breaths when there is not enough time is sufficient. Failure of the jaw to relax following the administration of suxamethonium should lead to the suspicion of malignant hyperpyrexia and the institution of a failed intubation drill followed by close observation.

Pinnock CA, Lin ES, Smith T. *Fundamentals of Anaesthesia*, 2nd Edn. Greenwich Medical Media Ltd, 2003, Section 1: Chapter 2

A **28.** **A.** true **B.** false **C.** false **D.** false **E.** true

Known triggers of malignant hyperpyrexia are all the inhalational agents including sevoflurane and desflurane, suxamethonium, possibly phenothiazines and some antidepressants. Agents thought to be safe include thiopentone, propofol, nitrous oxide, opioids, pancuronium, vecuronium, benzodiazepines, all local anaesthetics, neostigmine, glycopyrrolate, atropine, ephedrine and other vasopressors.

Pinnock CA, Lin ES, Smith T. *Fundamentals of Anaesthesia*, 2nd Edn. Greenwich Medical Media Ltd, 2003, Section 1: Chapter 3

A **29.** **A.** true **B.** false **C.** true **D.** false **E.** false

A homozygote for the atypical or silent gene will typically cause paralysis for 2–4 h. Low levels of plasma cholinesterase are seen in pregnancy, liver disease, renal failure and certain drug therapies (e.g. ecothiophate for glaucoma, monoamine oxidase inhibitors (MAOIs), neostigmine, pyridostigmine). Management of suxamethonium apnoea is supportive with sedation and ventilation until muscle function returns. FFP or heat-treated human plasma cholinesterase could be used but the condition is self-limiting and blood products have an inherent infection risk.

Pinnock CA, Lin ES, Smith T. *Fundamentals of Anaesthesia*, 2nd Edn. Greenwich Medical Media Ltd, 2003, Section 1: Chapter 3

A **30.** **A.** true **B.** true **C.** false **D.** false **E.** false

The sural nerve branches off the tibial nerve in the popliteal fossa. The saphenous nerve needs to be blocked in addition to a popliteal nerve block in order to provide complete anaesthesia of the leg below the knee. It supplies sensation to the medial aspect of the ankle and foot distally up to the metatarsophalangeal joint of the great toe. It can be blocked at the knee.

Pinnock CA, Fischer HBJ, Jones RP. *Peripheral Nerve Blockade*. Churchill Livingstone, 1996

A 31. A. false   **B.** true   **C.** false   **D.** false   **E.** true

The femoral nerve lies lateral to the femoral vessels. It divides into anterior and posterior divisions as it enters the leg under the inguinal ligament. The anterior division provides the motor supply to the sartorius and two sensory nerves innervating the anterior and medial aspects of the thigh including the skin overlying the knee. The posterior division provides motor fibres to quadriceps femoris, articular fibres to the knee joint and ends as the saphenous nerve supplying sensation to the medial aspect of the ankle and foot. Femoral nerve block alone requires 10–15 ml of local anaesthetic and is suitable for knee surgery but not for ankle surgery where sciatic nerve block is required in addition.

Pinnock CA, Fischer HBJ, Jones RP. *Peripheral Nerve Blockade*. Churchill Livingstone, 1996

A 32. A. true   **B.** false   **C.** true   **D.** false   **E.** true

The 5 letter code relates to the chamber paced (I), the chamber sensed (II), the response to sensed information (III), programmability/rate modulation (IV), antitachycardia functions (V). Ideally, bipolar diathermy should be used but unipolar may be used if absolutely necessary, providing the current pathway from instrument to plate is well away from the heart. In addition, short bursts followed by long pause should be used. Rate modulation and antitachycardia/defibrillator functions should be turned off prior to anaesthesia. Defibrillator paddles should be placed perpendicular to the direction of the pacing leads. Pacing boxes are designed to protect themselves by channelling current away from the box and down the lead – this may result in burns. The anterior external pacing paddle should be placed at the lower left sternal edge to minimise chest wall impedance caused by the pectoral muscles.

Mills SJ, Maguire SL, Barker JM. *The Clinical Anaesthesia Viva Book*. Greenwich Medical Media Ltd, 2002

A **33.** **A.** true   **B.** false   **C.** true   **D.** true   **E.** false

Clinical signs of inadequate depth of anaesthesia include increase in heart rate, increase in blood pressure, dilatation of the pupils, sweating, lacrimation and increase in metabolic rate. Guedel described the four stages of anaesthesia in unpremedicated patients breathing ether in air. Stage II (the excitatory phase) describes irregular breathing. Stage III is surgical anaesthesia.

Pinnock CA, Lin ES, Smith T. *Fundamentals of Anaesthesia*, 2nd Edn. Greenwich Medical Media Ltd, 2003, Section 1: Chapter 3

A **34.** **A.** true   **B.** true   **C.** false   **D.** false   **E.** true

Symptoms include pleuritic chest pain and dyspnoea. Signs include ipsilateral reduced expansion, increased percussion note, reduced breath sounds and reduced oxygen saturation. Tension pneumothorax may produce any of the above plus signs of mediastinal shift and cardiovascular embarrassment.

Mills SJ, Maguire SL, Barker JM. *The Clinical Anaesthesia Viva Book*. Greenwich Medical Media Ltd, 2002

A **35.** **A.** false   **B.** false   **C.** false   **D.** true   **E.** false

Inheritance was originally thought to be autosomal dominant but is now known to be more complex. 50% of families worldwide have been linked to the ryanodine receptor on chromosome 19. Most confirmed cases have had at least one previous uneventful anaesthesia. Known triggers include potent inhalational anaesthetic agents and suxamethonium – nitrous oxide is safe. Early features are a steep rise in $ETCO_2$ level and tachycardia. Temperature rise, which may eventually be extremely rapid, is not one of the early features.

Halsall PJ, Hopkins PM. Malignant hyperthermia. *BJA CEPD Review* Feb, 2003

A **36.** **A.** true   **B.** true   **C.** false   **D.** true   **E.** false

A ratio of mandibular length to posterior mandibular depth >3.6 predicts difficult intubation. Protruding incisors make intubation more difficult. Reduced distance from the C1 spinous process to the occiput is predictive of difficult intubation.

Pinnock CA, Lin ES, Smith T. *Fundamentals of Anaesthesia*, 2nd Edn. Greenwich Medical Media Ltd, 2003, Section 1: Chapter 1

A 37. **A.** true   **B.** true   **C.** false   **D.** true   **E.** false

Decontamination is the physical removal of infected material by washing or scrubbing. Disinfection is the killing of non-sporing organisms and sterilisation is the killing of all microorganisms including viruses, fungi and spores. Methods of disinfection include pasteurisation or chemicals such as gluteraldehyde, formaldehyde, 70% alcohol, chlorhexidine, 10% hypochlorite, hydrogen peroxide or phenol. Sterilisation can be achieved by dry heat at 150°C for 30 min, moist heat by steam under pressure, ethylene oxide or gamma radiation.

Pinnock CA, Lin ES, Smith T. *Fundamentals of Anaesthesia*, 2nd Edn. Greenwich Medical Media Ltd, 2003, Section 4: Chapter 3

A 38. **A.** false   **B.** true   **C.** true   **D.** false   **E.** true

Carbon monoxide binds to the alpha chain of haemoglobin and has 250 times the affinity of oxygen for this. Other criteria for HBO therapy include loss of consciousness at any time, neurological signs, cardiac ischaemia/arrhythmias and pregnancy. The half-life of COHb in air is 4–5 h.

Mills SJ, Maguire SL, Barker JM. *The Clinical Anaesthesia Viva Book*. Greenwich Medical Media Ltd, 2002

A 39. **A.** false   **B.** false   **C.** true   **D.** false   **E.** true

The inguinal ligament extends from the internal ring laterally to the external ring medially. The anterior wall is formed by the external and internal oblique muscles. The inguinal canal transmits the ilioinguinal nerve.

Pinnock CA, Lin ES, Smith T. *Fundamentals of Anaesthesia*, 2nd Edn. Greenwich Medical Media Ltd, 2003, Section 1: Chapter 10

A 40. **A.** false   **B.** true   **C.** true   **D.** true   **E.** false

The mucous membrane of the larynx below the vocal cords is supplied by the recurrent laryngeal nerve. Above the cords, the internal (sensory) laryngeal nerve provides the sensory supply.

All the muscles of the larynx are also supplied by the recurrent laryngeal nerve except cricothyroid which is supplied by the superior (or external) laryngeal nerve.

The arterial supply to the larynx arises from branches of the superior and inferior thyroid arteries.

Pinnock CA, Lin ES, Smith T. *Fundamentals of Anaesthesia*, 2nd Edn. Greenwich Medical Media Ltd, 2003, Section 1: Chapter 10

A 41. A. true **B.** false **C.** true **D.** true **E.** true

The sciatic nerve can be stretched between the sciatic notch and the head of the fibula. The saphenous nerve can be compressed against the medial tibial condyle. The obturator nerve can be damaged due to flexion at the obturator foramen. The femoral nerve can be injured if flexion of the thigh stretches the nerve against the inguinal ligament. Other nerves that can be damaged in this position are the posterior tibial nerve, the common peroneal nerve and the cervical spine.

Pinnock CA, Lin ES, Smith T. *Fundamentals of Anaesthesia*, 2nd Edn. Greenwich Medical Media Ltd, 2003, Section 1: Chapter 3

A 42. A. true **B.** true **C.** false **D.** false **E.** true

Massive blood transfusion can cause a metabolic acidosis for a number of reasons including: lactate from the red cells, citric acid (the anticoagulant in stored blood) and poor perfusion of the patient due to shock. Decreased plasma ionised calcium can be caused by citrate binding to calcium. Hyperkalaemia can be a problem because the potassium concentration in stored blood can reach 30 mmol/l after 3 weeks. Hyponatraemia is not generally seen with massive blood transfusion. Hypothermia is a frequent clinical problem as the stored blood is kept at 4°C.

Pinnock CA, Lin ES, Smith T. *Fundamentals of Anaesthesia*, 2nd Edn. Greenwich Medical Media Ltd, 2003, Section 1: Chapter 3

Mills SJ, Maguire SL, Barker JM. *The Clinical Anaesthesia Viva Book*. Greenwich Medical Media Ltd, 2002

A 43. **A.** false **B.** true **C.** false **D.** true **E.** true

Features of pure mitral stenosis on a chest X-ray include:

- Features of an enlarged left atrium
  - A double right heart border
  - Straightening of the upper left heart border
  - Splaying of the carina to more than 60°C
- Features of pulmonary hypertension and oedema
  - Upper lobe blood diversion
  - Prominent pulmonary arteries in perihilar regions but 'pruned' peripherally
  - Kerley B lines

The mitral valve annulus may be calcified.

Cardiomegaly would suggest the coexistence of mitral regurgitation.

Mills SJ, Maguire SL, Barker JM. *The Clinical Anaesthesia Viva Book*. Greenwich Medical Media Ltd, 2002

A 44. **A.** true **B.** true **C.** false **D.** true **E.** true

The trigeminal nerve is the largest cranial nerve and supplies sensory fibres to the scalp, face, mouth, teeth, nasal cavity and paranasal air sinuses. It supplies motor fibres to the muscles of mastication. The nerve has three main branches: the ophthalmic nerve, the maxillary nerve and the mandibular nerve. The soft palate is innervated by the greater and lesser palatine nerve branches of the maxillary nerve. The tympanic membrane is innervated on its outer surface by the auriculotemporal nerve, a branch of the mandibular nerve. The skin over the angle of the jaw is supplied by the great auricular nerve (C2 and C3) and not by the trigeminal nerve. The infraorbital nerve, a branch of the maxillary nerve, supplies the skin of the nose. The supraorbital nerve, a branch of the ophthalmic division, supplies the conjunctiva.

Pinnock CA, Lin ES, Smith T. *Fundamentals of Anaesthesia*, 2nd Edn. Greenwich Medical Media Ltd, 2003, Section 1: Chapter 10

Snell RS. *Clinical Anatomy for Medical Students*, 3rd Edn. Little, Brown and Co., 2000, Chapter 11

The use of premedication is controversial and not considered essential. Reactions typically begin 30–60 min after the start of the procedure. In patients with spina bifida, the incidence may be as high as 60%. Patients may show cross-reactivity with certain foods such as bananas, chestnuts and avocados. Anaphylaxis is a type I immediate hypersensitivity reaction.

Mills SJ, Maguire SL, Barker JM. *The Clinical Anaesthesia Viva Book.* Greenwich Medical Media Ltd, 2002

A 46. **A.** true   **B.** false   **C.** true   **D.** false   **E.** false

The right coronary artery arises from the anterior aortic sinus passing between the right atrium and pulmonary trunk to run in the right coronary sulcus to anastomose with the left coronary artery. The coronary sinus runs in the posterior atrio-ventricular groove and drains into the right atrium. The AV node and the atrioventricular bundle are supplied by the right coronary artery.

Pinnock CA, Lin ES, Smith T. *Fundamentals of Anaesthesia*, 2nd Edn. Greenwich Medical Media Ltd, 2003, Section 1: Chapter 10

Snell RS. *Clinical Anatomy for Medical Students*, 3rd Edn. Little, Brown and Co., 2000

A 47. **A.** true   **B.** true   **C.** false   **D.** true   **E.** false

SC disease has a less severe clinical course than sickle cell disease (SCD) but patients can suffer the same complications, especially in pregnancy when it can present. Many patients have hyposplenism (due to auto-splenectomy) and therefore antibiotic cover must be active against *Streptococcus pneumoniae*. Pain is a major problem with SCD patients and can be very severe, necessitating large doses of opioids. A crisis may be precipitated by cold, alcohol, stress, infection, dehydration and hypoxia among other things. HbS arises due to a single DNA base change which results in the substitution of valine for glutamic acid at position 6 of the beta chain.

Pinnock CA, Lin ES, Smith T. *Fundamentals of Anaesthesia*, 2nd Edn. Greenwich Medical Media Ltd, 2003, Section 2: Chapter 3

Mills SJ, Maguire SL, Barker JM. *The Clinical Anaesthesia Viva Book.* Greenwich Medical Media Ltd, 2002

A **48.** **A.** false **B.** false **C.** false **D.** false **E.** false

The epidural space is open laterally to the intervertebral foraminae. The epidural space lies outside of the dura mater. The space is closed superiorly at the foramen magnum and inferiorly at the sacrococcygeal membrane. The veins are valveless and form the venous plexus of Bateson communicating between the pelvic veins and cerebral veins.

Pinnock CA, Lin ES, Smith T. *Fundamentals of Anaesthesia*, 2nd Edn. Greenwich Medical Media Ltd, 2003, Section 1: Chapter 5, Section 2: Chapter 9

A **49.** **A.** true **B.** true **C.** false **D.** false **E.** true

Acute intermittent porphyria is the commonest of a rare group of inherited diseases of errors of metabolism that result in the accumulation of excessive amounts of porphyrins and their precursors. Many anaesthetic drugs increase porphyrin production and administration may result in neurotoxic porphyrin levels. Acute attacks commonly present with abdominal pain, nausea and vomiting and neuropsychiatric symptoms. Labile blood pressure, tachycardia and sweating also occur frequently. In AIP, there is excess production and urinary excretion of delta-ALA. Treatment is mainly supportive. Intravenous haematin appears to be of benefit and a high carbohydrate is maintained, which has an indirect effect on porphyrin overproduction.

Pinnock CA, Lin ES, Smith T. *Fundamentals of Anaesthesia*, 2nd Edn. Greenwich Medical Media Ltd, 2003, Section 3: Chapter 6

Craft TM, Upton PM. *Key Topics in Anaesthesia*, 2nd Edn. BIOS Scientific Publishers, 1995, p 229

A **50.** **A.** false **B.** true **C.** true **D.** true **E.** false

Haemolysis, elevated liver enzymes and low platelets (HELLP) syndrome is a severe form of pre-eclampsia that involves severe hepatic dysfunction. Oliguria is a more likely feature than polyuria.

Morgan GE, Mikhail MS. *Clinical Anaesthesiology*, 2nd Edn. Appleton and Lange, 1996, Chapter 43

Pinnock CA, Lin ES, Smith T. *Fundamentals of Anaesthesia*, 2nd Edn. Greenwich Medical Media Ltd, 2003, Section 1: Chapter 5

A 1. **A.** true **B.** false **C.** false **D.** false **E.** true

The knee jerk is a monosynaptic reflex which arises at L2 level in the spinal cord. The afferents arise from the quadriceps muscle, and higher centres have an effect which may be demonstrated.

Pinnock CA, Lin ES, Smith T. *Fundamentals of Anaesthesia*, 2nd Edn. Greenwich Medical Media Ltd, 2003, Section 2: Chapter 9

Snell RS. *Clinical Anatomy for Medical Students*, 3rd Edn. Little, Brown and Co., 2000, Chapter 5

A 2. **A.** true **B.** false **C.** false **D.** true **E.** false

Vertebrate myelinated fibres vary in diameter between 2 and 20 microns. At the neuromuscular junction transmission is chemical, the neurotransmitter being acetylcholine. Intrafusal muscle fibres are supplied by gamma-motor (efferent) neurones which are termed fusimotor.

Pinnock CA, Lin ES, Smith T. *Fundamentals of Anaesthesia*, 2nd Edn. Greenwich Medical Media Ltd, 2003, Section 2: Chapters 4, 9

A 3. **A.** false **B.** true **C.** false **D.** true **E.** true

The adrenal medullary vesicles secrete adrenaline, noradrenaline and dopamine. The catecholamines are stored in a complex bound to chromogranin. The vesicles contain the enzyme dopamine beta hydroxylase, which catalyses the formation of noradrenaline from dopamine. Release of catecholamines requires ATP for energy but the mechanism is first triggered by cholinergic preganglionic fibres in the greater splanchnic nerves. On stimulation, acetylcholine is released which then leads to an increase in sodium permeability which triggers an influx of calcium ions.

Vesicles are subsequently drawn to the cell membrane and fuse, releasing their contents by exocytosis.

Pinnock CA, Lin ES, Smith T. *Fundamentals of Anaesthesia*, 2nd Edn. Greenwich Medical Media Ltd, 2003, Section 2: Chapter 12

A 4. **A.** true **B.** true **C.** false **D.** true **E.** false

The speed of conduction along a nerve fibre is influenced by axon diameter and myelination. Conduction velocity increases as the axon diameter increases (motor fibres have a greater diameter than sensory). The myelin sheath results in an increased speed of conduction as the action potential jumps very rapidly from node to node through the axon that is insulated by the sheath. Changes in serum potassium concentration alter the ionic basis of membrane potential (dictated by the Nernst equation) and conduction is slowed if the serum potassium is low.

Pinnock CA, Lin ES, Smith T. *Fundamentals of Anaesthesia*, 2nd Edn. Greenwich Medical Media Ltd, 2003, Section 2: Chapter 9

A 5. **A.** true **B.** false **C.** false **D.** false **E.** false

Autonomic ganglia may involve several differing neurotransmitters. Those known to have an effect include: dopamine, acteylcholine and gonadotrophin releasing hormone (GnRH).

Pinnock CA, Lin ES, Smith T. *Fundamentals of Anaesthesia*, 2nd Edn. Greenwich Medical Media Ltd, 2003, Section 2: Chapter 9

A 6. **A.** false **B.** true **C.** true **D.** false **E.** false

Nerves are relatively poor conductors in a passive sense, conduction is an active self-propagating process. Large fibres are faster and maximum velocity of propagation is 120 m/s which is seen in A-alpha fibres (proprioception and motor). Pain is transmitted in A-delta (myelinated) and C-fibres (unmyelinated). The small C-fibres are more susceptible to the action of local anaesthetic drugs.

Pinnock CA, Lin ES, Smith T. *Fundamentals of Anaesthesia*, 2nd Edn. Greenwich Medical Media Ltd, 2003, Section 2: Chapter 9

A 7. **A.** true **B.** true **C.** true **D.** false **E.** false

The dorsal columns transmit fine touch and proprioception. Temperature and pain sensations travel in the contralateral spinothalamic tracts. Fine touch is transmitted in the posterior white column in the medial and lateral fasiculi, which each connect to their respective cuneate and gracile nuclei. The pyramidal tract is a descending (motor) tract. The posterior and anterior spinocerbellar tracts ascend in the lateral column and transmit proprioception to the cerebellum without crossing.

Pinnock CA, Lin ES, Smith T. *Fundamentals of Anaesthesia*, 2nd Edn. Greenwich Medical Media Ltd, 2003, Section 1: Chapter 10

A 8. **A.** true **B.** false **C.** true **D.** true **E.** false

Muscle spindles are stretch receptors in skeletal muscle. They initiate the reflex arc when stretched. The structure of spindles is fusiform, consisting of intrafusal fibres with type Ia and type II sensory afferents and gamma motor efferent fibres. A change in muscle tension may be as a result of direct contraction or passive stretching.

Pinnock CA, Lin ES, Smith T. *Fundamentals of Anaesthesia*, 2nd Edn. Greenwich Medical Media Ltd, 2003, Section 2: Chapter 4

A 9. **A.** true **B.** false **C.** false **D.** true **E.** true

The ionic basis of the membrane potential relies on the distribution of ions on each side of the cell membrane. In a nerve cell the concentration of potassium ions is much greater intracellularly than extracellularly (brought about by the sodium-potassium ATPase pump) and the Nernst equation can be applied to calculate the membrane potential for this individual ion. The Goldman constant-field equation is required to calculate the value of the overall membrane potential as it takes into account sodium, chloride and potassium. The inside of the cell is $-90\,mV$ with respect to the outside and this value is not a function of the diameter. During an action potential the polarity reverses, albeit briefly.

Pinnock CA, Lin ES, Smith T. *Fundamentals of Anaesthesia*, 2nd Edn. Greenwich Medical Media Ltd, 2003, Section 2: Chapter 5

10. **A.** true   **B.** true   **C.** true   **D.** false   **E.** false

The normal cell membrane is a lipid bi-layer construction which is impermeable to organic anions. It is freely permeable to water and small hydrophobic molecules such as oxygen and nitrogen can cross with ease. Larger uncharged molecules like glucose diffuse only slowly but active transport mechanisms exist to overcome this.

Pinnock CA, Lin ES, Smith T. *Fundamentals of Anaesthesia*, 2nd Edn. Greenwich Medical Media Ltd, 2003, Section 2: Chapter 1

A **11.** **A.** false   **B.** false   **C.** true   **D.** true   **E.** false

The initial phase of the action potential occurs when an increase in sodium conductance results in an influx of sodium ions thus raising the potential within the cell. The action potential is propagated in a linear fashion in unmyelinated fibres (although in myelinated fibres conduction jumps between nodes of Ranvier in a manner termed 'saltatory' conduction). Myelinated fibres transmit the action potential 50 times faster than unmyelinated fibres. During the action potential the voltage swing occurs between -70 and $+35\,$mV, a $105\,$mV difference.

Pinnock CA, Lin ES, Smith T. *Fundamentals of Anaesthesia*, 2nd Edn. Greenwich Medical Media Ltd, 2003, Section 2: Chapter 9

A **12.** **A.** true   **B.** false   **C.** true   **D.** false   **E.** true

Normal CSF has a volume of 150 ml total with a pH of around 7.32. It is iso-osmolar with plasma (290 mosm/kg water) and contains little protein at 0.3 g/l. The specific gravity of CSF lies around 1006 at 37°C.

Pinnock CA, Lin ES, Smith T. *Fundamentals of Anaesthesia*, 2nd Edn. Greenwich Medical Media Ltd, 2003, Section 2: Chapter 2

A **13.** **A.** false   **B.** false   **C.** true   **D.** true   **E.** false

Lymph is produced at a rate of 2–4 l in 24 h. The protein content of lymph is lower than that of plasma (although the extent varies

Physiology

Answers

between organs drained). Plasma lipids are carried in lymph as lipoproteins and chylomicrons. Lymph contains all the coagulation factors, antibodies and lymphocytes but red cells and platelets are rare.

Pinnock CA, Lin ES, Smith T. *Fundamentals of Anaesthesia*, 2nd Edn. Greenwich Medical Media Ltd, 2003, Section 2: Chapter 2

A **14.** **A.** true **B.** true **C.** false **D.** true **E.** false

The autonomic nervous system (ANS) comprises two portions, the sympathetic and parasympathetic systems. It is not under direct conscious control. The ANS supplies efferent and afferent paths with respect to the viscera. The parasympathetic system is also called the cranio-sacral outflow because it is derived from the cranial nerves (III, VII, IX and X) and the sacral segments S2–4. In contrast the sympathetic system arises from the roots T1–L2.

Pinnock CA, Lin ES, Smith T. *Fundamentals of Anaesthesia*, 2nd Edn. Greenwich Medical Media Ltd, 2003, Section 2: Chapter 9

A **15.** **A.** false **B.** true **C.** true **D.** true **E.** false

Pain is transmitted in the spinothalamic tracts. The transmission of pain at cord level may be modulated by opioid peptides, particularly dynorphin interneurones. It is known that descending pathways from the PAG area can block noxious afferent signals. The thalamus integrates pain signals before relaying them on to the somatosensory cortex. A-delta fibres terminate in Rexed lamina I and V of the dorsal horn, whereas small C-fibres terminate in laminae I and II.

Pinnock CA, Lin ES, Smith T. *Fundamentals of Anaesthesia*, 2nd Edn. Greenwich Medical Media Ltd, 2003, Section 2: Chapter 9

A **16.** **A.** false **B.** true **C.** true **D.** true **E.** false

The intraocular pressure (IOP) may be lowered by hypotension, values of less than 80 mmHg mean are accompanied by a fall in IOP but a rise in blood pressure is not necessarily accompanied by a proportional rise in IOP. Coughing, sneezing and head down tilt result in increase in IOP. The angle of the anterior chamber affects the drainage of aqueous humor and drainage is increased when the ciliary muscle contracts, conversely relaxation of the ciliary muscle in an eye which has a narrow anterior angle may impede drainage and cause raised IOP.

Craft TM, Upton PM. *Key Topics in Anaesthesia*, 2nd Edn. BIOS Scientific Publishers, 1995, p 197

A 17. **A.** true **B.** false **C.** true **D.** false **E.** false

The withdrawal reflex is an example of a polysynaptic reflex in response to a noxious stimulus. The initial response is flexor contraction and extensor inhibition of the limb. With increasing strength of stimulus there will also be extension of the opposing limb (in animals the response may spread to all four limbs). The withdrawal reflex may be slowed or partially suppressed by higher centres. The mass reflex is a profound withdrawal extension pattern of all four limbs accompanied by visceral effects seen in the paraplegic state after application of a minor noxious stimulus.

Pinnock CA, Lin ES, Smith T. *Fundamentals of Anaesthesia*, 2nd Edn. Greenwich Medical Media Ltd, 2003, Section 2: Chapter 9

A 18. **A.** false **B.** false **C.** false **D.** true **E.** false

Both sympathetic and parasympathetic systems have a similar structure with both pre- and postganglionic fibres. Transmission at autonomic ganglia is primarily cholinergic. Dopamine via D2 receptors is involved to a lesser extent as is GnRH. The grey rami communicantes connect ganglia to their effector targets in the relevant spinal segments. Sympathetic preganglionic neurones leave the spinal cord at levels T1 to L2 and pass via the white rami communicantes to ganglia of the sympathetic chain.

Pinnock CA, Lin ES, Smith T. *Fundamentals of Anaesthesia*, 2nd Edn. Greenwich Medical Media Ltd, 2003, Section 1: Chapter 10, Section 2: Chapter 9

A 19. **A.** false **B.** false **C.** false **D.** true **E.** true

Sudden depolarisation produces an action potential. The inside of the cell becomes increasingly positive due to a sharp rise in the sodium conductance which is transient. Three factors limit depolarisation speed, first the temporary opening of the sodium channels, secondly with increasing intracellular electropositivity the initial sodium gradient reduces, and finally there is an increase in potassium conductance.

Pinnock CA, Lin ES, Smith T. *Fundamentals of Anaesthesia*, 2nd Edn. Greenwich Medical Media Ltd, 2003, Section 2: Chapter 9

A 20. **A.** false **B.** true **C.** false **D.** true **E.** false

Normal body temperature is tightly regulated to within 0.2° of 37°C. Shivering is a reflex controlled by the hypothalamus which has a temperature regulating centre (the thalamus is not involved). Brown fat may release fatty acids after oxidation, an action mediated by the adrenergic system. Certain endogenous factors are known to be pyrogenic. These include interleukins, interferons and tumour necrosis factor. Normal body temperature shows diurnal variation with a peak in the afternoon and a trough at night.

Pinnock CA, Lin ES, Smith T. *Fundamentals of Anaesthesia*, 2nd Edn. Greenwich Medical Media Ltd, 2003, Section 2: Chapter 11

A 21. **A.** true **B.** true **C.** true **D.** false **E.** false

The control of arterial tone is alpha adrenoceptor mediated, and concerns noradrenaline as the transmitter. Sympathectomy, having removed any sympathetic vessel tone, results in vasodilatation and an increase in flow. The response to cold and haemorrhage is an increase in vasoconstriction.

Pinnock CA, Lin ES, Smith T. *Fundamentals of Anaesthesia*, 2nd Edn. Greenwich Medical Media Ltd, 2003, Section 2: Chapter 6

A 22. **A.** true **B.** true **C.** false **D.** false **E.** true

Acetylcholine is a neurotransmitter found in the cerebral cortex, thalamus and limbic system. It is likely to be associated with memory, perception and cognitive function. Serotonin is associated with the limbic system and neocortex. Dopamine has a role in the hypothalamus (not the thalamus) in the regulation of prolactin secretion. Noradrenaline is a neurotransmitter in the cerebellum and the locus ceruleus and the hypothalamus.

Pinnock CA, Lin ES, Smith T. *Fundamentals of Anaesthesia*, 2nd Edn. Greenwich Medical Media Ltd, 2003, Section 2: Chapter 9

A **23.** **A.** true **B.** true **C.** false **D.** true **E.** true

Water intoxication is associated with general and progressive signs of cerebral irritation followed by depression. Confusion, delirium, nausea and vomiting progress to convulsions and coma. Plasma sodium falls in a dilutional manner so hyponatraemia is seen.

Pinnock CA, Lin ES, Smith T. *Fundamentals of Anaesthesia*, 2nd Edn. Greenwich Medical Media Ltd, 2003, Section 2: Chapter 2

A **24.** **A.** true **B.** true **C.** true **D.** true **E.** false

The oxygen content of blood is calculated by adding together the amount of oxygen carried by haemoglobin and the amount of oxygen carried in solution. In states of anaemia the former is reduced, as it is in methaemoglobinaemia and in the presence of carboxyhaemoglobin. Dissolved oxygen only represents about 1% of the total and is a function of pO_2. It therefore increases under hyperbaric conditions.

Pinnock CA, Lin ES, Smith T. *Fundamentals of Anaesthesia*, 2nd Edn. Greenwich Medical Media Ltd, 2003, Section 2: Chapter 8

A **25.** **A.** false **B.** true **C.** false **D.** false **E.** true

Left ventricular end diastolic pressure (LVEDP) correlates closely with left ventricular end diastolic volume and therefore provides an index of left ventricular preload. LVEDP will be raised when compliance of the ventricle is reduced. Raised LVEDP increases myocardial work and therefore oxygen requirement. It is increased in aortic regurgitation because regurgitant blood re-enters the ventricle thus raising LVEDP on a chronic basis.

Morgan GE, Mikhail MS. *Clinical Anaesthesiology*, 2nd Edn. Appleton and Lange, 1996, Chapter 19

Pinnock CA, Lin ES, Smith T. *Fundamentals of Anaesthesia*, 2nd Edn. Greenwich Medical Media Ltd, 2003, Section 2: Chapter 5

A 26. A. true **B.** true **C.** false **D.** true **E.** true

Iodine is converted to iodide in the body. Iodide is essential for the synthesis of thyroid hormones. Several organs in the body can concentrate iodide against a concentration gradient. These include the breast, stomach and salivary glands. Iodine is added to some brands of salt on sale. High concentrations of iodides decrease thyroid activity and especially its blood supply. Therefore iodides are frequently prescribed before surgery to decrease the vascularity of the gland.

Guyton AC. *Textbook of Medical Physiology*, 7th Edn. WB Saunders, 1986, Chapter 76

A 27. A. false **B.** false **C.** true **D.** false **E.** false

Haemoglobin is a molecule comprised of four polypeptide chains, two alpha and two beta. Each haemoglobin molecule carries four molecules of oxygen. Each polypeptide chain contains a porphyrin ring with a ferrous ion at its centre.

Pinnock CA, Lin ES, Smith T. *Fundamentals of Anaesthesia*, 2nd Edn. Greenwich Medical Media Ltd, 2003, Section 2: Chapter 3

A 28. A. false **B.** true **C.** false **D.** true **E.** true

The monosynaptic stretch reflex occurs when the muscle is stretched passively. An example is the stretching of the quadriceps muscle by a tap on the patellar tendon. The knee jerk sensory fibre is a Ia fibre which synapses with an alpha motor neurone at the level of L2. It is independent of higher centres although it can be influenced by activity in higher centres. Transection of the cord is followed by a variable degree of spinal shock where all reflexes are depressed or absent. Recovery of reflexes may take up to 6 weeks.

Pinnock CA, Lin ES, Smith T. *Fundamentals of Anaesthesia*, 2nd Edn. Greenwich Medical Media Ltd, 2003, Section 2: Chapter 9

A **29.** **A.** true **B.** true **C.** false **D.** true **E.** false

All the figures quoted are an average for each tissue measured in ml per 100 g of tissue. The correct answer for whole body is 8.6 and for skin is 12.8. These figures may vary widely under different circumstances.

Pinnock CA, Lin ES, Smith T. *Fundamentals of Anaesthesia*, 2nd Edn. Greenwich Medical Media Ltd, 2003, Section 2: Chapter 6

A **30.** **A.** true **B.** false **C.** true **D.** true **E.** false

The molecular weight of myoglobin is 17,000 while that of haemoglobin is 64,450. A myoglobin molecule combines with only one molecule of oxygen, the oxygen dissociation curve being a rectangular hyperbola to the left of the haemoglobin dissociation curve. The Bohr effect does not occur and there is no combination with carbon dioxide.

Pinnock CA, Lin ES, Smith T. *Fundamentals of Anaesthesia*, 2nd Edn. Greenwich Medical Media Ltd, 2003, Section 2: Chapter 3

A **31.** **A.** false **B.** false **C.** true **D.** false **E.** false

Carbon dioxide combines with haemoglobin to form carbamino-haemoglobin. Increased carbon dioxide in the blood shifts the oxyhaemoglobin dissociation curve to the right (the Bohr effect). Carbon dioxide enters erythrocytes and combines with water to from carbonic acid. The subsequent dissociation into hydrogen and bicarbonate ions leads to bicarbonate ions leaving the cell and chloride ions entering – the chloride shift. 10% of carbon dioxide transport is carried in dissolved form. It is more soluble in the blood than oxygen.

Pinnock CA, Lin ES, Smith T. *Fundamentals of Anaesthesia*, 2nd Edn. Greenwich Medical Media Ltd, 2003, Section 2: Chapter 8

West JB. *Respiratory Physiology – The Essentials*, 5th Edn. Williams & Wilkins, 1995, Chapter 6

A 32. **A.** false **B.** false **C.** true **D.** true **E.** false

Cardiac output is decreased on standing from supine due to decreased venous return as a result of venous pooling in the legs. The diminished baroreceptor excitation reflexly increases the heart rate and increases the strength of contraction to compensate. Metabolic demand causes increases in cardiac output mainly mediated via the sympathetic nervous system. This applies to eating and exercise. In hypothermia there is bradycardia and a fall in cardiac output.

Berne RM, Levy MN. *Cardiovascular Physiology*, 7th Edn. Mosby, 1997, Chapter 9

A 33. **A.** false **B.** true **C.** true **D.** true **E.** true

Factors which shift the oxyhaemoglobin dissociation curve to the right include: higher temperature, acidosis, increased pCO_2 and raised 2,3-DPG levels. The curve for foetal haemoglobin lies to the left of adult. A right shift of the curve facilitates 'unloading' of oxygen. In the pulmonary capillaries a left shift of the curve occurs.

Pinnock CA, Lin ES, Smith T. *Fundamentals of Anaesthesia*, 2nd Edn. Greenwich Medical Media Ltd, 2003, Section 2: Chapter 8

A 34. **A.** false **B.** false **C.** false **D.** false **E.** false

Gastric emptying is increased by mechanical distension, gastrin and parasympathetic activity. Fat and protein are slower to leave the stomach than carbohydrate. Gastric emptying is inhibited by sympathetic activity and the presence of acid or fat in the duodenum.

Pinnock CA, Lin ES, Smith T. *Fundamentals of Anaesthesia*, 2nd Edn. Greenwich Medical Media Ltd, 2003, Section 2: Chapter 10

A **35.** **A.** false **B.** true **C.** true **D.** false **E.** false

In the normal heart atrial contraction is a significant factor in ventricular filling. Coronary blood flow is greatest in diastole and increases in hypoxia. In the phase of isovolumetric relaxation the AV valves are shut and no ventricular filling occurs. The bundle of Kent is an accessory conducting bundle not present in the normal heart.

Pinnock CA, Lin ES, Smith T. *Fundamentals of Anaesthesia*, 2nd Edn. Greenwich Medical Media Ltd, 2003, Section 2: Chapters 5, 6

A **36.** **A.** true **B.** false **C.** false **D.** false **E.** false

The right vagus is mainly distributed to the SA node and the left vagus mainly to the AV node. Vagal stimulation affects rate rather than filling, thus producing bradycardia. Coronary blood flow averages 250 ml/min in the resting state. Stroke volume is related to end diastolic filling pressure (and volume) which is affected by the length of the previous diastole.

Pinnock CA, Lin ES, Smith T. *Fundamentals of Anaesthesia*, 2nd Edn. Greenwich Medical Media Ltd, 2003, Section 2: Chapter 5

A **37.** **A.** false **B.** false **C.** true **D.** true **E.** false

The Fick principle states that the amount of a substance taken up by an organ (or the whole of the body) per unit time, is equal to the arterial concentration of the substance minus the venous concentration, times the blood flow.

Pinnock CA, Lin ES, Smith T. *Fundamentals of Anaesthesia*, 2nd Edn. Greenwich Medical Media Ltd, 2003, Section 2: Chapter 5

A **38.** **A.** false **B.** true **C.** true **D.** true **E.** true

An increase in preload will increase LVEDV and therefore stroke volume and consequently cardiac output and arterial blood pressure. Stimulation of atrial stretch receptors causes the release of atrial natriuretic peptide (ANP) which has a diuretic action. The direction of change in heart rate is governed by the balance between the Bainbridge reflex and the baroreceptor reflex. If the blood volume is reduced then the baroreceptor reflex will predominate.

Berne RM, Levy MN. *Cardiovascular Physiology*, 7th Edn. Mosby, 1997, Chapter 4

Pinnock CA, Lin ES, Smith T. *Fundamentals of Anaesthesia*, 2nd Edn. Greenwich Medical Media Ltd, 2003, Section 2: Chapter 5

A 39. A. false **B.** false **C.** true **D.** true **E.** true

Fibrin and thrombin are formed from their inactive forms, fibrinogen and prothrombin respectively. Plasminogen is converted to plasmin as part of the fibrinolysis cascade. Christmas factor is factor IX. Antihaemophilic factor is factor VIII, a co-factor in the coagulation cascade.

Hoffbrand AV, Pettit JE. *Essential Haematology*, 3rd Edn. Blackwell Science, 1993, Chapter 16

Pinnock CA, Lin ES, Smith T. *Fundamentals of Anaesthesia*, 2nd Edn. Greenwich Medical Media Ltd, 2003, Section 2: Chapter 3

A 40. A. true **B.** true **C.** false **D.** false **E.** false

The waves in the JVP are:
- The 'a' wave is atrial contraction.
- The 'c' wave is isovolumetric contraction.
- The 'x' descent reflects the fall in right ventricular pressure when the pulmonary valve opens.
- The 'v' wave is due to the build-up of pressure in the atrium until the tricuspid valve opens.
- The 'y' descent is the following drop in pressure caused by rapid ventricular filling when the tricuspid valve opens.
- Only the 'x' descent is prominent in cardiac tamponade.

Pinnock CA, Lin ES, Smith T. *Fundamentals of Anaesthesia*, 2nd Edn. Greenwich Medical Media Ltd, 2003, Section 2: Chapter 5

A 41. A. true **B.** false **C.** false **D.** false **E.** false

Pulmonary vascular resistance falls markedly as the lungs expand and fill with air. This decreases pulmonary artery pressures and increases blood flow to the left atrium. Umbilical vessels constrict and placental circulation ceases resulting in increased systemic vascular resistance and arterial pressure. Left atrial pressure becomes higher than right atrial pressure and this closes the foramen ovale. The ductus arteriosus closes functionally soon after birth (usually within 24 h) due to exposure to oxygenated blood and reduced prostaglandin-E2. The first breath generates a negative pressure of about 50 cmH$_2$O.

Pinnock CA, Lin ES, Smith T. *Fundamentals of Anaesthesia*, 2nd Edn. Greenwich Medical Media Ltd, 2003, Section 2: Chapter 14

A 42. **A.** false   **B.** true   **C.** false   **D.** true   **E.** false

Transection of the spinal cord is followed by a period of spinal shock during which all reflex responses are profoundly depressed. This usually lasts between 2 and 6 weeks.

Pinnock CA, Lin ES, Smith T. *Fundamentals of Anaesthesia*, 2nd Edn. Greenwich Medical Media Ltd, 2003, Section 2: Chapter 9

A 43. **A.** false   **B.** true   **C.** false   **D.** true   **E.** true

Testing for Hepatitis C was introduced in 1991 and the incidence of post transfusion Hepatitis C is probably now less than 1:30,000.

DIC, which has low fibrinogen as a feature, can occur with an incompatible blood transfusion. Congestive cardiac failure is a common complication of blood transfusion, especially in the elderly.

Pinnock CA, Lin ES, Smith T. *Fundamentals of Anaesthesia*, 2nd Edn. Greenwich Medical Media Ltd, 2003, Section 2: Chapter 3

Handbook of Transfusion Medicine, 2nd Edn. HMSO, 1996, Chapter 5

A 44. **A.** true   **B.** true   **C.** false   **D.** true   **E.** false

The importance of the bicarbonate buffer system is due to the ease of excretion of CO$_2$ by the lungs and the continuous maintenance of buffer base levels through reabsorption of bicarbonate in the kidneys. Haemoglobin has 6 times the buffering capacity of the plasma proteins due to its abundance and the dissociation of the imidazole groups on the 38 histidine residues on each molecule. The phosphate buffer system is extremely important intracellularly.

Pinnock CA, Lin ES, Smith T. *Fundamentals of Anaesthesia*, 2nd Edn. Greenwich Medical Media Ltd, 2003, Section 2: Chapter 7

A **45.** **A.** true **B.** true **C.** true **D.** true **E.** true

Amniotic fluid embolus is a rare and often fatal condition whose features include all these plus hypotension and DIC.

Pinnock CA, Lin ES, Smith T. *Fundamentals of Anaesthesia*, 2nd Edn. Greenwich Medical Media Ltd, 2003, Section 1: Chapter 5

A **46.** **A.** true **B.** true **C.** true **D.** true **E.** false

Pinnock CA, Lin ES, Smith T. *Fundamentals of Anaesthesia*, 2nd Edn. Greenwich Medical Media Ltd, 2003, Section 2: Chapter 9

A **47.** **A.** false **B.** true **C.** true **D.** false **E.** true

Between 1.0 and 1.5 l of saliva are produced each day with a pH of about 6.5. Intrinsic factor is a mucoprotein essential for the absorption of vitamin B12. It is secreted by parietal cells in the stomach. The pancreas produces about 1,500 ml of alkaline fluid (pH 8.0) per day, which consists of digestive enzymes secreted by the acina and bicarbonate produced by the epithelial cells of the ducts.

Pinnock CA, Lin ES, Smith T. *Fundamentals of Anaesthesia*, 2nd Edn. Greenwich Medical Media Ltd, 2003, Section 2: Chapter 10

A **48.** **A.** false **B.** true **C.** false **D.** false **E.** false

A mixed peripheral nerve contains lower motor neurones. Cut nerve fibres are capable of regeneration but this takes time. After traumatic lesion of a peripheral nerve there is total loss of cutaneous sensibility and interruption of postganglionic sympathetic fibres results in a loss of vascular control and the skin becomes red and hot at first. The chances of a mixed nerve recovering well are much less than those of a pure sensory or motor nerve.

Snell RS. *Clinical Anatomy for Medical Students*, 3rd Edn. Little, Brown and Co., 2000, Chapter 4

A 49. A. false **B.** true **C.** true **D.** true **E.** false

Glucose supply to the brain is a priority in starvation as it is largely dependent on glucose as an energy substrate. The brain can however metabolise ketones. As metabolism switches to the burning of fats the respiratory quotient drops towards 0.7. Glucagon levels go up as the body enters a catabolic phase with increased glycogenolysis. Increased protein breakdown leads to increased urinary nitrogen excretion. The accumulation of acetyl CoA leads to ketoacidosis, not alkalosis.

Pinnock CA, Lin ES, Smith T. *Fundamentals of Anaesthesia*, 2nd Edn. Greenwich Medical Media Ltd, 2003, Section 2: Chapter 11

A 50. A. false **B.** true **C.** true **D.** true **E.** false

Primary active transport requires energy from ATP. Secondary active transport does not require energy directly.

Pinnock CA, Lin ES, Smith T. *Fundamentals of Anaesthesia*, 2nd Edn. Greenwich Medical Media Ltd, 2003, Section 2: Chapters 1, 7, 10

A 51. A. true **B.** false **C.** false **D.** false **E.** false

The ECF is approximately one-third of total body water. The Fick principle is used to measure blood flow. Magnesium and potassium reside mainly intracellularly. ECF can be measured with radioactive inulin.

Pinnock CA, Lin ES, Smith T. *Fundamentals of Anaesthesia*, 2nd Edn. Greenwich Medical Media Ltd, 2003, Section 2: Chapter 2

A 52. A. true **B.** true **C.** true **D.** false **E.** true

Cortisol exerts a direct negative feedback control with inhibition of both CRH and ACTH release. Over 90% of cortisol is transported combined with a plasma globulin but only about 50% of aldosterone is protein bound. Adrenal androgens are secreted in both sexes but their effects are very minor.

Pinnock CA, Lin ES, Smith T. *Fundamentals of Anaesthesia*, 2nd Edn. Greenwich Medical Media Ltd, 2003, Section 2: Chapter 12

A 53. A. false **B.** true **C.** false **D.** true **E.** true

Myocardial relaxation is a metabolically active phase when calcium re-uptake occurs by the sarcoplasmic reticulum. Catecholamines aid this process and cause more isovolumetric relaxation per unit time. Atrial contraction contributes up to 25% of ventricular filling in the normal heart. The vast majority of coronary blood flow occurs during diastole. Diastasis is the slow ventricular filling phase of diastole. There is only a small increase in ventricular volume during this time.

Pinnock CA, Lin ES, Smith T. *Fundamentals of Anaesthesia*, 2nd Edn. Greenwich Medical Media Ltd, 2003, Section 2: Chapter 5

A 54. A. true **B.** false **C.** true **D.** true **E.** true

The ductus arteriosus closes as a result of exposure to oxygenated blood and reduced prostaglandin E2 production. The ductus venosus shunts oxygenated blood from the umbilical vein (SaO_2 of 80%) through the liver to the IVC. The majority of this mixed IVC blood (SaO_2 of 65%) is directed through the foramen ovale to the brain and upper body. SVC blood is directed preferentially through the right ventricle, pulmonary artery and the left side of the heart. The right ventricle is dominant in the foetal circulation and possesses a thicker ventricular wall at the time of birth. The mixed aortic and ductal blood flow supplies the lower body with blood with a saturation of 55%.

Pinnock CA, Lin ES, Smith T. *Fundamentals of Anaesthesia*, 2nd Edn. Greenwich Medical Media Ltd, 2003, Section 2: Chapter 14

A 55. A. false **B.** true **C.** true **D.** false **E.** false

Red blood cell mass increases by 30% and plasma volume increases by 50% causing an dilutional anaemia (physiological)

with a haematocrit decrease of 15%. Iodine uptake by the thyroid gland increases. Thyroid binding globulin levels double but free plasma T3 and T4 levels remain normal.

Pinnock CA, Lin ES, Smith T. *Fundamentals of Anaesthesia*, 2nd Edn. Greenwich Medical Media Ltd, 2003, Section 2: Chapter 13

A **56.** **A.** true **B.** true **C.** false **D.** true **E.** true

Blood flow is greatest to the most dependent parts of the lung because of gravitational effects. Gravity also affects the distribution of ventilation because of the variation in intrapleural pressure. This pressure will be greater in the lower lung and therefore will lie on a different part of the compliance curve to the upper lung. The alveoli in the lower lung are less distended and therefore are on a steeper part of the compliance curve. Greater expansion will occur here than in the already more distended alveoli of the upper lung. The upper and lower lungs will have different V/Q ratios. The greater the blood flow in relation to the ventilation, the more the blood gases for that area of the lung will tend towards a mixed venous blood gas picture (i.e. high CO_2 and low O_2). As ventilation increases in relation to blood flow the gases will tend towards inspired gas (i.e. high O_2 and low CO_2).

Pinnock CA, Lin ES, Smith T. *Fundamentals of Anaesthesia*, 2nd Edn. Greenwich Medical Media Ltd, 2003, Section 2: Chapter 8

West JB. *Respiratory Physiology – The Essentials*, 5th Edn. Williams & Wilkins, 1995, Chapter 5

A **57.** **A.** false **B.** true **C.** true **D.** true **E.** false

Pinnock CA, Lin ES, Smith T. *Fundamentals of Anaesthesia*, 2nd Edn. Greenwich Medical Media Ltd, 2003, Section 2: Chapter 6

A **58.** **A.** true **B.** true **C.** false **D.** false **E.** false

The normal oxygen content of arterial blood is about 20 ml/100 ml of blood and that of mixed venous blood is about 15 ml/100 ml of blood giving a saturation of about 75%. This gives an average O_2 consumption of 5 ml/100 ml of blood.

The figures for kidney, brain and heart are 1.4, 6.2 and 11.4 ml/100 ml of blood respectively. The liver receives a large part of its blood supply from the portal vein which contains blood that is already largely deoxygenated.

Fundamentals of Anaesthesia, Section 2: Chapter 6

A 59. A. true **B.** false **C.** true **D.** true **E.** true

Most postganglionic sympathetic neurones are noradrenergic but those that supply sweat glands, piloerector muscles and a few blood vessels are cholinergic.

Pinnock CA, Lin ES, Smith T. *Fundamentals of Anaesthesia*, 2nd Edn. Greenwich Medical Media Ltd, 2003, Section 2: Chapter 9

A 60. A. false **B.** true **C.** true **D.** true **E.** false

Carbohydrates, acids and fat in the duodenum (not the oesophagus) reduce gastric emptying. Secretin is released in response to a low pH in the duodenum. It causes release of bicarbonate rich fluid from the pancreas.

Pinnock CA, Lin ES, Smith T. *Fundamentals of Anaesthesia*, 2nd Edn. Greenwich Medical Media Ltd, 2003, Section 2: Chapter 10

A 61. A. false **B.** false **C.** true **D.** true **E.** false

Release of aldosterone is the result of secretion of renin from the granular cells in the juxtaglomerular apparatus. Causes of this are low body sodium content and low extracellular volume. The mechanisms by which release of renin occurs are increased sympathetic activity (decreased ECV will cause low cardiac output), decreased wall tension in the arterioles at the granular cells and decreased NaCl delivery to the macula densa mechanism.

Pinnock CA, Lin ES, Smith T. *Fundamentals of Anaesthesia*, 2nd Edn. Greenwich Medical Media Ltd, 2003, Section 2: Chapter 7

A 62. **A.** false **B.** false **C.** false **D.** true **E.** true

The dorsal columns carry ipsilateral touch, vibration and proprioception signals. The lateral spinothalamic tract conveys pain and temperature. Allodynia is a painful response to a normally non-painful stimulus. Hyperalgesia is an increased response to a normally painful stimulus.

Neuropathic pain can be caused by development of abnormal communication between the sympathetic nervous system and the sensory nervous system. The gate theory of pain suggests that simultaneous stimulation of other modalities within the same spinal segment can reduce pain sensation (e.g. T.E.N.S).

Morgan GE, Mikhail MS. *Clinical Anaesthesiology*, 2nd Edn. Appleton and Lange, 1996, Chapter 18

Pinnock CA, Lin ES, Smith T. *Fundamentals of Anaesthesia*, 2nd Edn. Greenwich Medical Media Ltd, 2003, Section 2: Chapter 9

A 63. **A.** false **B.** true **C.** false **D.** false **E.** false

Prolactin, Growth hormone, ACTH and TSH are all synthesised in the anterior pituitary.

Pinnock CA, Lin ES, Smith T. *Fundamentals of Anaesthesia*, 2nd Edn. Greenwich Medical Media Ltd, 2003, Section 2: Chapter 12

A 64. **A.** false **B.** true **C.** false **D.** true **E.** true

Insulin promotes potassium entry into cells and is used therapeutically for this purpose. Insulin is the body's main anabolic hormone and as such it increases glycogen synthesis.

Pinnock CA, Lin ES, Smith T. *Fundamentals of Anaesthesia*, 2nd Edn. Greenwich Medical Media Ltd, 2003, Section 2: Chapter 12

A 65. **A.** true **B.** false **C.** true **D.** true **E.** true

Glucagon stimulates insulin release.

Pinnock CA, Lin ES, Smith T. *Fundamentals of Anaesthesia*, 2nd Edn. Greenwich Medical Media Ltd, 2003, Section 2: Chapter 12

A **66.** **A.** true **B.** false **C.** true **D.** true **E.** true

Thyroid hormones are bound to thyroglobulin for storage.
Circulating hormones are bound to thyroid binding globulin.
Radioactive iodine uptake is an index of thyroid function.
Carbimazole may cause goitre as a result of increased TSH
secretion stimulated by the decline in circulating thyroid
hormones.

Pinnock CA, Lin ES, Smith T. *Fundamentals of Anaesthesia*, 2nd Edn.
Greenwich Medical Media Ltd, 2003, Section 2: Chapter 12

A **67.** **A.** true **B.** true **C.** true **D.** true **E.** false

The chemoreceptors respond primarily to a reduction in arterial
oxygen tension, but are also sensitive to a rise in arterial pCO_2
tension or a fall in pH. The chemoreceptors have a very high
oxygen consumption in order to act as oxygen delivery sensors
to the brain.

Pinnock CA, Lin ES, Smith T. *Fundamentals of Anaesthesia*, 2nd Edn.
Greenwich Medical Media Ltd, 2003, Section 2: Chapters 6, 8

A **68.** **A.** false **B.** false **C.** false **D.** true **E.** false

CSF is produced by modified ultrafiltration. The glucose level
is about two-thirds that of plasma. The cerebral aqueduct
connects the third ventricle to the fourth ventricle.

Pinnock CA, Lin ES, Smith T. *Fundamentals of Anaesthesia*, 2nd Edn.
Greenwich Medical Media Ltd, 2003, Section 2: Chapter 2

Snell RS. *Clinical Anatomy for Medical Students*, 3rd Edn. Little, Brown
and Co., 2000, Chapter 13

A **69.** **A.** false **B.** true **C.** false **D.** false **E.** false

Surfactant is a phospholipid based substance which increases
lung compliance by reducing surface tension. Surfactant is
depleted after interruption of blood flow.

Pinnock CA, Lin ES, Smith T. *Fundamentals of Anaesthesia*, 2nd Edn.
Greenwich Medical Media Ltd, 2003, Section 2: Chapter 8

West JB. *Respiratory Physiology – The Essentials*, 5th Edn. Williams & Wilkins,
1995, Chapter 7

A **70.** **A.** true   **B.** true   **C.** true   **D.** true   **E.** true

This is a question about positive end expiratory pressure (PEEP). PEEP increases mean intrathoracic pressure which will reduce preload (volume) but increase the CVP (pressure). It increases pulmonary vascular resistance and reduces cardiac output. PEEP is used to increase the FRC, decrease shunt and therefore increase arterial O_2 tension.

Hinds CJ, Watson D. *Intensive Care – A Concise Textbook*. WB Saunders, 1995, Chapter 13

A **71.** **A.** true   **B.** true   **C.** true   **D.** true   **E.** false

Snell RS. *Clinical Anatomy for Medical Students*, 3rd Edn. Little, Brown and Co., 2000, Chapter 4

A **72.** **A.** true   **B.** true   **C.** true   **D.** false   **E.** false

Sympathetic activity causes relaxation of bronchial smooth muscle. Sympathetic stimulation of the radial muscle of the iris causes mydriasis. Parasympathetic fibres constitute the efferent limb of the voiding reflex. Sympathetic activity decreases motility and tone in the intestine.

Pinnock CA, Lin ES, Smith T. *Fundamentals of Anaesthesia*, 2nd Edn. Greenwich Medical Media Ltd, 2003, Section 2: Chapter 9

A **73.** **A.** false   **B.** false   **C.** false   **D.** true   **E.** true

The gamma efferent system supplies skeletal muscle spindles. If gamma efferent tone is high then slight disturbances in skeletal muscle length elicit reflex contraction. Clinically this is manifest as hypertonicity. Conversely, when tone is low, hypotonicity results.

Pinnock CA, Lin ES, Smith T. *Fundamentals of Anaesthesia*, 2nd Edn. Greenwich Medical Media Ltd, 2003, Section 2: Chapter 4

A **74.** **A.** false   **B.** false   **C.** true   **D.** false   **E.** true

The magnitude of the membrane potential depends on the distributions of sodium, chloride and potassium ions and the membrane permeability to these ions. The Goldman constant-field equation incorporates all of these and is used to calculate membrane potential. The Nernst equation calculates the magnitude of the equilibrium potential for a given ion. The resting membrane potential of a neuron is about $-70\,mV$. Chloride flux is governed by the concentration gradient and the electrical gradient. The intracellular free calcium concentration is much lower than in the ECF.

Pinnock CA, Lin ES, Smith T. *Fundamentals of Anaesthesia*, 2nd Edn. Greenwich Medical Media Ltd, 2003, Section 2: Chapter 9

A 75. A. true **B.** false **C.** true **D.** true **E.** true

Pain sensations are relayed via the spinothalamic tracts to the thalamus. Beta endorphin is a member of a family of opioid peptides that produce analgesia. It is released during exercise. The Gate theory explains why non-painful stimuli in the same area can cause analgesia.

Pinnock CA, Lin ES, Smith T. *Fundamentals of Anaesthesia*, 2nd Edn. Greenwich Medical Media Ltd, 2003, Section 2: Chapter 9

A 76. A. true **B.** true **C.** false **D.** true **E.** true

Clinically this would cause a Horner's syndrome, the features of which are constriction of the pupil, drooping of the upper eyelid, nasal congestion and enophthalmos. The loss of sympathetic tone would cause arterial vasodilatation. The lacrimal glands are under parasympathetic control.

Morgan GE, Mikhail MS. *Clinical Anaesthesiology*, 2nd Edn. Appleton and Lange, 1996, Chapter 18

A 77. A. true **B.** false **C.** true **D.** false **E.** false

Portal venous pressure is about 10 mmHg. Portal venous blood flow represents 70% of the liver's blood supply, however about 50% of the oxygen delivery is from the hepatic artery. Portal vein oxygen saturation is about 85%.

Pinnock CA, Lin ES, Smith T. *Fundamentals of Anaesthesia*, 2nd Edn. Greenwich Medical Media Ltd, 2003, Section 2: Chapter 6

A. true   **B.** true   **C.** true   **D.** false   **E.** true

GH mobilises free fatty acids and decreases glucose uptake into cells and increases hepatic glucose output. In common with insulin it promotes protein synthesis.

Pinnock CA, Lin ES, Smith T. *Fundamentals of Anaesthesia*, 2nd Edn. Greenwich Medical Media Ltd, 2003, Section 2: Chapter 12

A 79. **A.** true   **B.** true   **C.** true   **D.** true   **E.** true

Activation of the renin-angiotensin system is caused by reductions in ECF, blood pressure or plasma sodium. As a result angiotensin II levels increase and stimulate aldosterone secretion. Increases in plasma potassium concentration also stimulate aldosterone secretion. ADH is released in response to surgical stress, leading to aldosterone secretion.

Pinnock CA, Lin ES, Smith T. *Fundamentals of Anaesthesia*, 2nd Edn. Greenwich Medical Media Ltd, 2003, Section 2: Chapters 7, 12

A 80. **A.** true   **B.** true   **C.** true   **D.** true   **E.** true

Secretion of PTH, a polypeptide, is directly stimulated by decreased plasma calcium concentration. PTH stimulates calcium release from bone, increases the rate of calcium reabsorption from the renal tubules, increases urinary phosphate excretion and increased the rate at which vitamin D is converted to the active form.

Pinnock CA, Lin ES, Smith T. *Fundamentals of Anaesthesia*, 2nd Edn. Greenwich Medical Media Ltd, 2003, Section 2: Chapter 12

A 81. **A.** true   **B.** false   **C.** false   **D.** true   **E.** false

The carotid bodies have the highest tissue blood flow per 100 g in the body. The carotid bodies are chemoreceptors (not baroceptors) that respond to changes in pO_2 (not oxygen content), pCO_2 and pH. Complete loss of hypoxic ventilatory drive has been shown in patients with bilateral carotid body resection.

Pinnock CA, Lin ES, Smith T. *Fundamentals of Anaesthesia*, 2nd Edn. Greenwich Medical Media Ltd, 2003, Section 2: Chapter 8

West JB. *Respiratory Physiology – The Essentials*, 5th Edn. Williams & Wilkins, 1995, Chapter 8

Physiology

Answers

A 82. **A.** false **B.** true **C.** false **D.** true **E.** true

Hyperventilation will cause a respiratory alkalosis and consequently the urinary pH will increase in attempt to correct this. Mild degrees of hypoxia will cause sympathetic stimulation with a consequent increase in heart rate and cardiac output. Alkalosis causes increased affinity of Hb for oxygen due to the shift of the oxygen-haemoglobin dissociation curve. Erythropoietin is secreted in response to hypoxia but its effect is not seen acutely.

Pinnock CA, Lin ES, Smith T. *Fundamentals of Anaesthesia*, 2nd Edn. Greenwich Medical Media Ltd, 2003, Section 2: Chapters 3, 8

A 83. **A.** false **B.** false **C.** true **D.** false **E.** false

Type II pneumocytes produce surfactant under the influence of cortisol from 26 weeks gestation. The oxygen saturation in the descending aorta is about 58% and the saturation in the ductus arteriosus is about 52%. This is because the more oxygenated blood from the IVC is directed across the foramen ovale into the aorta. The heavily deoxygenated blood from the SVC is directed through the right side of the heart (mixed with some more oxygenated blood from the IVC) and most of this will cross the ductus arteriosus. Blood flow through the ductus ceases shortly after birth due to exposure to oxygenated blood. Umbilical venous blood has a higher pO_2 than the umbilical artery.

Case RM. *Variations in Human Physiology*. Manchester University Press, 1985, Chapter 2

Pinnock CA, Lin ES, Smith T. *Fundamentals of Anaesthesia*, 2nd Edn. Greenwich Medical Media Ltd, 2003, Section 2: Chapter 14

A 84. **A.** true **B.** true **C.** true **D.** false **E.** false

Systolic blood pressure increases relatively more than the diastolic. Stroke volume is increased in mild to moderate exercise. Potassium is lost in the sweat especially in humid conditions. Renal blood flow is decreased to as little as 30% of normal.

Pinnock CA, Lin ES, Smith T. *Fundamentals of Anaesthesia*, 2nd Edn. Greenwich Medical Media Ltd, 2003, Section 2: Chapter 6

A **85.** **A.** true **B.** true **C.** false **D.** true **E.** true

The renal cortex receives the majority of renal blood flow. Renal blood flow is autoregulated between mean arterial pressures of 90 and 200 mmHg. Most anaesthetic agents reduce renal blood flow.

Pinnock CA, Lin ES, Smith T. *Fundamentals of Anaesthesia*, 2nd Edn. Greenwich Medical Media Ltd, 2003, Section 2: Chapter 7

A **86.** **A.** true **B.** true **C.** true **D.** true **E.** true

During exercise, the first four situations arise in the muscles.

Pinnock CA, Lin ES, Smith T. *Fundamentals of Anaesthesia*, 2nd Edn. Greenwich Medical Media Ltd, 2003, Section 2: Chapter 8

A **87.** **A.** false **B.** false **C.** true **D.** true **E.** true

The blood-brain barrier consists of the ultrafiltration barrier in the choroid plexuses and the barrier around cerebral capillaries. Water, CO_2 and O_2 diffuse freely across but the transport of glucose is controlled, as are many other substances. Permeability is altered if the barrier is inflamed. This fact is used in the treatment of meningitis when otherwise some antibiotics may not cross the blood-brain barrier. The barrier develops during the early years of life and this explains why bile pigments are able to damage the neonatal brain if they become very jaundiced.

Pinnock CA, Lin ES, Smith T. *Fundamentals of Anaesthesia*, 2nd Edn. Greenwich Medical Media Ltd, 2003, Section 2: Chapter 6

A **88.** **A.** true **B.** false **C.** false **D.** true **E.** true

The JVP is conventionally measured with the patient reclined at 45 degrees. The 'a' wave is absent in atrial fibrillation because there is no atrial contraction.

Pinnock CA, Lin ES, Smith T. *Fundamentals of Anaesthesia*, 2nd Edn. Greenwich Medical Media Ltd, 2003, Section 2: Chapter 5

A 89. **A.** true **B.** false **C.** false **D.** false **E.** false

During the Valsalva manoeuvre (forced expiration against a closed glottis) there is decreased venous return and therefore a decrease in cardiac output (apart from a small increase initially as blood from the lungs is pushed back to the left atrium). Diminished baroreceptor stimulation causes a tachycardia and increased systemic vascular resistance.

Pinnock CA, Lin ES, Smith T. *Fundamentals of Anaesthesia*, 2nd Edn. Greenwich Medical Media Ltd, 2003, Section 2: Chapter 6

A 90. **A.** false **B.** false **C.** true **D.** false **E.** false

The 'a' wave is atrial contraction. The 'c' wave is due to bulging of the tricuspid valve during isovolumetric contraction. Cannon waves (giant 'a' waves) are classically seen in complete heart block as the atria contract against a closed tricuspid valve due to AV dissociation.

Pinnock CA, Lin ES, Smith T. *Fundamentals of Anaesthesia*, 2nd Edn. Greenwich Medical Media Ltd, 2003, Section 2: Chapter 5

A 91. **A.** false **B.** false **C.** false **D.** true **E.** true

Sodium and urea concentrations are higher in the plasma. CSF is more acidic (more hydrogen ions) due to the higher pCO_2.

Pinnock CA, Lin ES, Smith T. *Fundamentals of Anaesthesia*, 2nd Edn. Greenwich Medical Media Ltd, 2003, Section 2: Chapter 2

A 92. **A.** true **B.** false **C.** false **D.** false **E.** false

70% of CO_2 is carried as bicarbonate, 22% as carbamino compounds (mainly combined with haemoglobin) and 8% in solution.

Pinnock CA, Lin ES, Smith T. *Fundamentals of Anaesthesia*, 2nd Edn. Greenwich Medical Media Ltd, 2003, Section 2: Chapter 8

A 93. **A.** true **B.** true **C.** false **D.** false **E.** false

Muscles of inspiration are the external intercostals, the diaphragm, the scalene muscles and the sternomastoids.

West JB. *Respiratory Physiology – The Essentials*, 5th Edn. Williams & Wilkins, 1995, Chapter 7

A 94. **A.** false **B.** false **C.** true **D.** true **E.** false

This monosynaptic reflex is initiated by the muscle spindles which are in the muscle, not the tendon.

Pinnock CA, Lin ES, Smith T. *Fundamentals of Anaesthesia*, 2nd Edn. Greenwich Medical Media Ltd, 2003, Section 2: Chapter 9

A 95. **A.** true **B.** false **C.** true **D.** true **E.** true

Blood pressure rises briefly initially as the increased intrathoracic pressure is transmitted to the aorta. Cardiac output also increases slightly at this time as more blood is forced back to the left side of the heart from the lungs. A fall in blood pressure then occurs as venous return is impeded and cardiac output drops. This produces a reflex tachycardia and increased systemic vascular resistance.

Pinnock CA, Lin ES, Smith T. *Fundamentals of Anaesthesia*, 2nd Edn. Greenwich Medical Media Ltd, 2003, Section 2: Chapter 6

A 96. **A.** false **B.** false **C.** false **D.** false **E.** true

Renal plasma flow is the total amount of fluid (discounting the solid red blood cells) entering the kidney that is potentially filterable and is about 600 ml/min. Glomerular filtration rate (GFR) is the amount that is actually filtered and is about 125 ml/min. The filtration fraction is therefore 120/600 or 20%.

Pinnock CA, Lin ES, Smith T. *Fundamentals of Anaesthesia*, 2nd Edn. Greenwich Medical Media Ltd, 2003, Section 2: Chapter 7

A 97. **A.** false **B.** false **C.** true **D.** true **E.** true

Hypoxia causes hyperventilation with a subsequent respiratory alkalosis. Chronic hypoxia leads to increased secretion of erythropoietin and therefore a rising haematocrit.

Pinnock CA, Lin ES, Smith T. *Fundamentals of Anaesthesia*, 2nd Edn. Greenwich Medical Media Ltd, 2003, Section 2: Chapter 8

A **98.** **A.** true   **B.** false   **C.** false   **D.** false   **E.** false

The CSF contains very little protein (IgG is a protein), is about 150 ml in volume and flows around the structures of the CNS.

Pinnock CA, Lin ES, Smith T. *Fundamentals of Anaesthesia*, 2nd Edn. Greenwich Medical Media Ltd, 2003, Section 2: Chapter 2

A **99.** **A.** true   **B.** true   **C.** false   **D.** true   **E.** true

The aortic bodies are found along the arch of the aorta. The carotid sinus houses the baroreceptors and is an enlargement of the internal carotid artery just above its origin. The central chemoreceptors are located beneath the ventral surface of the medulla in the CNS.

Pinnock CA, Lin ES, Smith T. *Fundamentals of Anaesthesia*, 2nd Edn. Greenwich Medical Media Ltd, 2003, Section 2: Chapter 8

A **100.** **A.** false   **B.** true   **C.** true   **D.** false   **E.** true

In starvation, glycogenolysis occurs and the liver begins to use fatty acids as a source of energy. As the glycogen is depleted, gluconeogenesis increases using amino acids from the breakdown of muscle protein. Glycerol can be used to produce glucose but the free fatty acids undergo beta-oxidation to produce ATP in the mitochondria. Most tissues, including the brain, can ultimately adapt to the use of ketone bodies as a fuel source. However the brain cannot survive without glucose.

Pinnock CA, Lin ES, Smith T. *Fundamentals of Anaesthesia*, 2nd Edn. Greenwich Medical Media Ltd, 2003, Section 2: Chapter 11

A **101.** **A.** true   **B.** false   **C.** true   **D.** false   **E.** false

Potassium tends to diffuse out of cells against an electrical gradient. The resting membrane potential of a nerve fibre is about $-70\,mV$ and this changes by 105 mV to $+35\,mV$ during an action potential.

Pinnock CA, Lin ES, Smith T. *Fundamentals of Anaesthesia*, 2nd Edn. Greenwich Medical Media Ltd, 2003, Section 2: Chapter 9

A **102. A.** true **B.** false **C.** false **D.** true **E.** false

The T wave begins at the beginning of phase 3 of repolarisation where potassium permeability rapidly increases to restore the membrane potential. The T wave represents ventricular repolarisation and occurs during ventricular contraction. The P wave represents atrial systole. The first heart sound represents the closing of the AV valves and occurs early during ventricular contraction.

Pinnock CA, Lin ES, Smith T. *Fundamentals of Anaesthesia*, 2nd Edn. Greenwich Medical Media Ltd, 2003, Section 2: Chapter 5

A **103. A.** false **B.** false **C.** false **D.** false **E.** true

The average thickness of the respiratory membrane (which includes more than the alveolar wall) is 0.6 microns. The pores of Kohn are connections between alveoli. Alveoli have a diameter of about 0.3 mm. Alveolar type II cells produce surfactant.

Pinnock CA, Lin ES, Smith T. *Fundamentals of Anaesthesia*, 2nd Edn. Greenwich Medical Media Ltd, 2003, Section 2: Chapter 8

A **104. A.** true **B.** true **C.** false **D.** true **E.** true

The afferent nerve fibres from the carotid bodies pass through Hering's nerves to the glossopharyngeal nerves. The effect of CO_2 and hydrogen ion concentration on the peripheral chemoreceptors is much less than the direct effects of both these factors on the respiratory centre itself. The glomus cells of the carotid bodies contain large amounts of dopamine.

Pinnock CA, Lin ES, Smith T. *Fundamentals of Anaesthesia*, 2nd Edn. Greenwich Medical Media Ltd, 2003, Section 2: Chapter 6

West JB. *Respiratory Physiology – The Essentials*, 5th Edn. Williams & Wilkins, 1995, Chapter 8

A **105. A.** false **B.** true **C.** true **D.** false **E.** true

The central chemoreceptors are highly sensitive to changes in hydrogen ion concentration in the CSF (which is affected by bicarbonate), but are relatively insensitive to hypoxia.

Stimulation of peripheral chemoreceptors occurs up to five times more quickly than the central effect.

Pinnock CA, Lin ES, Smith T. *Fundamentals of Anaesthesia*, 2nd Edn. Greenwich Medical Media Ltd, 2003, Section 2: Chapters 6, 8

West JB. *Respiratory Physiology – The Essentials*, 5th Edn. Williams & Wilkins, 1995, Chapter 8

A 106. A. true **B.** true **C.** true **D.** true **E.** false

Anatomical dead space increases with large inspirations and also depends on the posture of the subject. Fowler's method of measuring anatomical dead space uses a rapid nitrogen analyser after a vital capacity breath of 100% O_2. Bohr's method is for calculating physiological dead space.

Pinnock CA, Lin ES, Smith T. *Fundamentals of Anaesthesia*, 2nd Edn. Greenwich Medical Media Ltd, 2003, Section 2: Chapter 8

West JB. *Respiratory Physiology – The Essentials*, 5th Edn. Williams & Wilkins, 1995, Chapter 2

A 107. A. true **B.** true **C.** false **D.** false **E.** false

ST segment depression and T wave flattening are both common in pregnancy and of little clinical significance. The SVR is reduced due to low-resistance vascular beds and the vasodilatory effects of oestrogens and progesterone. A third heart sound is common in pregnancy.

Pinnock CA, Lin ES, Smith T. *Fundamentals of Anaesthesia*, 2nd Edn. Greenwich Medical Media Ltd, 2003, Section 2: Chapter 13

A 108. A. false **B.** true **C.** true **D.** true **E.** false

The molecular weight of myosin is 480,000. The globular head of the myosin has ATP and actin binding sites.

Pinnock CA, Lin ES, Smith T. *Fundamentals of Anaesthesia*, 2nd Edn. Greenwich Medical Media Ltd, 2003, Section 2: Chapter 4

A 109. A. true **B.** true **C.** true **D.** true **E.** false

Sympathetic vasoconstrictor fibres supply the hepatic artery and the smooth muscle in the walls of the intrahepatic portal vein radicles.

Fundamentals of Anaesthesia, Section 2: Chapter 6

A **110.** **A.** false   **B.** true   **C.** true   **D.** true   **E.** true

In order to measure GFR a substance should also be: not secreted, not metabolised, not stored and easy to measure.

Fundamentals of Anaesthesia, Section 2: Chapter 7

A **111.** **A.** true   **B.** false   **C.** true   **D.** true   **E.** false

Normal creatinine clearance is 125 ml/min. This value remains remarkably constant day to day.

Pinnock CA, Lin ES, Smith T. *Fundamentals of Anaesthesia*, 2nd Edn. Greenwich Medical Media Ltd, 2003, Section 2: Chapter 7

A **112.** **A.** true   **B.** true   **C.** false   **D.** false   **E.** false

The extracellular fluid volume is about 14 l in an adult and represents about 20% of body weight. The ECF volume remains fairly constant throughout life when expressed as an index of body surface area.

Pinnock CA, Lin ES, Smith T. *Fundamentals of Anaesthesia*, 2nd Edn. Greenwich Medical Media Ltd, 2003, Section 2: Chapter 2

A **113.** **A.** true   **B.** false   **C.** true   **D.** false   **E.** true

The tubular maximum is independent of the blood glucose level but varies for different tubules. Most glucose is reabsorbed in the proximal tubule but more distal parts of the tubule are capable of reabsorption.

Pinnock CA, Lin ES, Smith T. *Fundamentals of Anaesthesia*, 2nd Edn. Greenwich Medical Media Ltd, 2003, Section 2: Chapter 7

A **114.** **A.** true   **B.** false   **C.** true   **D.** true   **E.** true

Pain signals are carried by the lateral spinothalamic tract.

Pinnock CA, Lin ES, Smith T. *Fundamentals of Anaesthesia*, 2nd Edn. Greenwich Medical Media Ltd, 2003, Section 2: Chapter 9

A **115.** **A.** true   **B.** true   **C.** true   **D.** false   **E.** true

It is worth remembering that an exercising muscle needs more oxygen unloading at tissue level and this is achieved by a right shift of the curve due to acidosis, increased pCO$_2$, increased concentration of 2,3-DPG and increased temperature. COHb shifts the curve to the left.

Pinnock CA, Lin ES, Smith T. *Fundamentals of Anaesthesia*, 2nd Edn. Greenwich Medical Media Ltd, 2003, Section 2: Chapter 8

A **116. A.** true **B.** true **C.** false **D.** true **E.** false

The ABO blood group is the most important because of the presence of naturally occurring IgM antibodies to groups A and B in subjects lacking these antigens. Only 3% of people in the UK have both of these antigens. 47% have neither (Group O). 80% of individuals can secrete ABO substances in their saliva and other bodily secretions. Rhesus D antibodies are IgG and this is clinically important because they can cross the placenta to cause haemolytic disease of the newborn. Kell and Duffy autoantibodies are clinically important because they are frequently responsible for transfusion reactions.

Pinnock CA, Lin ES, Smith T. *Fundamentals of Anaesthesia*, 2nd Edn. Greenwich Medical Media Ltd, 2003, Section 2: Chapter 3

A **117. A.** false **B.** true **C.** true **D.** false **E.** true

In moderate exercise, the cardiac output increases largely due to an increased heart rate. Increased pCO$_2$ stimulates the vasomotor centre to cause increased vasoconstriction, heart rate and stroke volume. Cardiac output may increase up to 7 times in a trained athlete. Cardiac output falls with IPPV because the raised intrathoracic pressure inhibits venous return.

Pinnock CA, Lin ES, Smith T. *Fundamentals of Anaesthesia*, 2nd Edn. Greenwich Medical Media Ltd, 2003, Section 2: Chapter 6

A **118. A.** false **B.** true **C.** false **D.** true **E.** true

FRC is the volume of gas remaining in the lungs at the end of a normal expiration. Residual volume is the amount remaining after a maximal expiration.

Pinnock CA, Lin ES, Smith T. *Fundamentals of Anaesthesia*, 2nd Edn. Greenwich Medical Media Ltd, 2003, Section 2: Chapter 8

119. **A.** false   **B.** false   **C.** true   **D.** false   **E.** true

GFR may be estimated by inulin clearance. PAH is used to measure renal plasma flow, which is usually about 600 ml/min. Sodium reabsorption requires energy (in the form of ATP) to establish an ionic gradient across the nephron cell membranes.

Pinnock CA, Lin ES, Smith T. *Fundamentals of Anaesthesia*, 2nd Edn. Greenwich Medical Media Ltd, 2003, Section 2: Chapter 7

120. **A.** true   **B.** true   **C.** false   **D.** true   **E.** false

The peripheral chemoreceptors respond to a decrease in pO_2 and pH, and an increase in pCO_2. Baroreceptors respond to a decrease in blood pressure. Doxapram also stimulates the respiratory centre. Hering's nerves are the afferent nerves from the carotid bodies to the glossopharyngeal nerves.

Pinnock CA, Lin ES, Smith T. *Fundamentals of Anaesthesia*, 2nd Edn. Greenwich Medical Media Ltd, 2003, Section 2: Chapter 8, Section 3: Chapter 13

121. **A.** true   **B.** true   **C.** true   **D.** true   **E.** false

Nociceptors are the sensory receptors for pain, and are naked nerve endings that exist in almost all tissues of the body. The receptors respond to different types of stimuli. Chemical stimuli are released in response to inflammation, e.g. bradykinin, H^+, substance P, histamine and K^+ ions. Purinergic receptors are a subtype of receptor which are stimulated by adenosine and its metabolites.

Pinnock CA, Lin ES, Smith T. *Fundamentals of Anaesthesia*, 2nd Edn. Greenwich Medical Media Ltd, 2003, Section 2: Chapter 9

122. **A.** true   **B.** true   **C.** true   **D.** false   **E.** true

The functions of the liver are myriad but include: the formation of bile, protein metabolism, carbohydrate metabolism, lipid metabolism, detoxification and excretion. The liver does not manufacture antibodies. This is the

Physiology

Answers

job of plasma cells. Acetylation is a conjugative phase 2 reaction.

Pinnock CA, Lin ES, Smith T. *Fundamentals of Anaesthesia*, 2nd Edn. Greenwich Medical Media Ltd, 2003, Section 2: Chapter 11

A 123. **A.** true **B.** true **C.** true **D.** false **E.** false

The neuroendocrine stress response causes increased secretion of catecholamines, ACTH, glucocorticoids, glucagon, thyroxine, angiotensin, aldosterone, GH, ADH and TSH. The response is mediated via the hypothalamus. ACTH causes release of aldosterone and glucocorticoids. Aldosterone increases sodium reabsorption in the distal tubule and increases potassium excretion. The actions of the glucocorticoids and glucagon include increased protein catabolism and increased hepatic glycogenolysis and gluconeogenesis. Protein catabolism causes a negative nitrogen balance.

Morgan GE, Mikhail MS. *Clinical Anaesthesiology*, 2nd Edn. Appleton and Lange, 1996, Chapter 50

Pinnock CA, Lin ES, Smith T. *Fundamentals of Anaesthesia*, 2nd Edn. Greenwich Medical Media Ltd, 2003, Section 2: Chapter 12

A 124. **A.** true **B.** false **C.** true **D.** false **E.** true

The anterior pituitary secretes ACTH, TSH, FSH, LH, prolactin and GH. The posterior pituitary secretes vasopressin (ADH) and oxytocin.

Pinnock CA, Lin ES, Smith T. *Fundamentals of Anaesthesia*, 2nd Edn. Greenwich Medical Media Ltd, 2003, Section 2: Chapter 12

A 125. **A.** false **B.** true **C.** false **D.** true **E.** false

Expiration is usually passive. The muscles of expiration are the abdominals and the internal intercostals. The internal intercostals pull the ribs down and inward.

West JB. *Respiratory Physiology – The Essentials*, 5th Edn. Williams & Wilkins, 1995, Chapter 7

Answers

A 126. **A.** true **B.** false **C.** true **D.** true **E.** false

Coronary blood flow at rest is about 250 ml/min and its main
determinant is aortic root diastolic pressure. The majority of
coronary blood flow occurs during diastole and therefore,
because diastole shortens with increasing heart rate, coronary
blood flow can become compromised with tachyarrhythmias.
Metabolic demands act to increase or decrease the oxygen
supply if demand is varied. Potassium and adenosine may be
responsible.

Pinnock CA, Lin ES, Smith T. *Fundamentals of Anaesthesia*, 2nd Edn.
Greenwich Medical Media Ltd, 2003, Section 2: Chapter 6

A 127. **A.** true **B.** true **C.** true **D.** true **E.** false

Hypomagnesaemia is common and often asymptomatic.
Weakness and electrical irritability of the heart may be
encountered. Hypomagnesaemia is frequently associated with
hypocalcaemia and any prolongation of the QT interval may
be a reflection of this. Magnesium has been used as emergency
treatment for Torsades de pointes (caused by prolongation
of the QT interval). Increased renal losses due to drug toxicity
(e.g. aminoglycosides) can cause hypomagnesaemia.

Morgan GE, Mikhail MS. *Clinical Anaesthesiology*, 2nd Edn. Appleton and
Lange, 1996, Chapter 28

A 128. **A.** true **B.** true **C.** false **D.** true **E.** true

Mean cerebral blood flow is about 55 ml/100 g/min and varies
between the different anatomical structures. The grey matter
may receive 70 ml/100 g/min while the white matter receives
30 ml/100 g/min. Arterial CO_2 tensions have a marked influence
over cerebral blood flow – much more than the pO_2. Cerebral
blood flow is autoregulated over a wide range of mean arterial
pressures, from about 60 mmHg to 160 mmHg. Adenosine and
potassium have both been implicated in adjusting local cerebral
perfusion.

Pinnock CA, Lin ES, Smith T. *Fundamentals of Anaesthesia*, 2nd Edn.
Greenwich Medical Media Ltd, 2003, Section 2: Chapter 6

A **129.** **A.** true **B.** true **C.** false **D.** true **E.** false

Haemorrhage results in decreased pulse pressure, increased heart rate and contractility and vasoconstriction and venoconstriction. On standing, the baroreceptors sense a decrease in blood pressure and activation of the sympathetic nervous system causes increased secretion of noradrenaline from the adrenal glands. This causes vasoconstriction. During exercise there is decreased systemic vascular resistance. Blood pressure is maintained due to the increased cardiac output. Increased intrathoracic pressure during the Valsalva manoeuvre causes decreased venous return and hence a decreased cardiac output. The baroreceptor response triggers vasoconstriction to maintain blood pressure. Increased ambient temperature causes vasodilatation to help the body lose heat.

Pinnock CA, Lin ES, Smith T. *Fundamentals of Anaesthesia*, 2nd Edn. Greenwich Medical Media Ltd, 2003, Section 2: Chapters 6, 12

A **130.** **A.** false **B.** true **C.** true **D.** false **E.** true

Dopamine is unaffected by the lung. 80% of bradykinin is inactivated while serotonin and prostaglandin E2 are almost completely removed. Angiotensin I is converted to angiotensin II by angiotensin converting enzyme (ACE) in the lung.

West JB. *Respiratory Physiology – The Essentials*, 5th Edn. Williams & Wilkins, 1995, Chapter 4

A **131.** **A.** true **B.** true **C.** true **D.** false **E.** false

The concentrations in mmol/l are given in the following table:

	Extracellular	*Intracellular*
Sodium	145	10
Chloride	117	3
Magnesium	1	4

ATP is synthesised inside the mitochondria and is used to provide energy inside the cells. Phosphate is one of the principal intracellular anions.

Pinnock CA, Lin ES, Smith T. *Fundamentals of Anaesthesia*, 2nd Edn. Greenwich Medical Media Ltd, 2003, Section 2: Chapter 2

A **132.** **A.** true **B.** false **C.** true **D.** true **E.** false

In the presence of ADH the collecting tubule wall is permeable to water, so the hypertonic medulla leads to the osmotic abstraction of water from the tubule. The medullary collecting tubules also become permeable to urea which leaves the tubule to contribute towards the osmolality of the renal medulla. ADH has no effect on the proximal tubule. ADH is synthesised in the supra optic nucleus of the hypothalamus and transported to the posterior pituitary within the nerve fibres.

Pinnock CA, Lin ES, Smith T. *Fundamentals of Anaesthesia*, 2nd Edn. Greenwich Medical Media Ltd, 2003, Section 2: Chapter 7

A **133.** **A.** false **B.** true **C.** false **D.** false **E.** true

Factor Va is the cofactor for the final conversion of prothrombin to thrombin by Factor Xa. Calcium is an important cofactor for many of the reactions in the coagulation cascade. Factor VII plays a central role in the extrinsic pathway and Factor VIII has a role in the intrinsic pathway.

Pinnock CA, Lin ES, Smith T. *Fundamentals of Anaesthesia*, 2nd Edn. Greenwich Medical Media Ltd, 2003, Section 2: Chapter 3

A **134.** **A.** false **B.** true **C.** false **D.** false **E.** true

Insulin is secreted by beta cells in the pancreas. Many agents regulate the secretion of insulin but the main ones are: increased plasma glucose concentration, increased amino acid concentrations, somatostatin secretion (which inhibits its release) and glucagon.

Pinnock CA, Lin ES, Smith T. *Fundamentals of Anaesthesia*, 2nd Edn. Greenwich Medical Media Ltd, 2003, Section 2: Chapter 12

A **135.** **A.** true **B.** false **C.** true **D.** false **E.** false

The vast majority of glucose reabsorption takes place in the proximal tubule, but more distal parts of the nephron are capable of reabsorbing glucose. No glucose is excreted in the urine unless the plasma glucose concentration is greater than 11 mmol/l. The proximal tubular glucose absorption is linked to sodium reabsorption by symporter carrier proteins that possess binding sites for both molecules.

Pinnock CA, Lin ES, Smith T. *Fundamentals of Anaesthesia*, 2nd Edn. Greenwich Medical Media Ltd, 2003, Section 2: Chapter 7

A 136. **A.** true **B.** true **C.** true **D.** true **E.** true

Hyperventilation due to a low FiO_2 is the primary response initiated by the chemoreceptors. The low pCO_2 produced leaves more room in the alveoli for O_2 (alveolar gas equation). Further features of acclimatisation include:

- Polycythaemia due to increased erythropoietin secretion
- Increased 2,3-DPG causing right shift of the oxyhaemoglobin dissociation curve
- Increased capillary density
- Increased mitochondrial density
- Increased concentration of respiratory enzymes
- Increased pulmonary artery pressures due to hypoxic vasoconstriction

Pinnock CA, Lin ES, Smith T. *Fundamentals of Anaesthesia*, 2nd Edn. Greenwich Medical Media Ltd, 2003, Section 2: Chapter 8

A 137. **A.** false **B.** true **C.** false **D.** true **E.** true

The basal metabolic rate (BMR) for an average young adult is about 70–100 kcal/h. Emotional states alter the BMR. Temperature does affect the BMR but the curve is U-shaped. If the environmental temperature drops for example, then heat conserving mechanisms such as shivering are activated, and the BMR rises. The metabolic rate rises with recent ingestion of food and therefore it is a condition that when measuring the BMR the subject must be starved for 12 h.

Pinnock CA, Lin ES, Smith T. *Fundamentals of Anaesthesia*, 2nd Edn. Greenwich Medical Media Ltd, 2003, Section 2: Chapter 11

A 138. **A.** true **B.** true **C.** false **D.** true **E.** true

The relationship between preload and contractility is described by the Frank–Starling relationship. Increased intracellular calcium levels increase contractility because more calcium is available to take part in excitation-contraction coupling. This same phenomenon explains the relationship between heart rate and contractility (the Bowditch phenomenon) in that the faster the heart rate the less time for intracellular calcium to be re-sequestered.

Pinnock CA, Lin ES, Smith T. *Fundamentals of Anaesthesia*, 2nd Edn. Greenwich Medical Media Ltd, 2003, Section 2: Chapter 5

A 139. A. true   **B.** true   **C.** true   **D.** true   **E.** true

Cardiac output is the product of heart rate and stroke volume. The later is determined by preload, contractility and afterload. Contractility is directly affected by the sympathetic nervous system.

Pinnock CA, Lin ES, Smith T. *Fundamentals of Anaesthesia*, 2nd Edn. Greenwich Medical Media Ltd, 2003, Section 2: Chapter 5

A 140. A. false   **B.** false   **C.** true   **D.** false   **E.** false

Transection of the spinal cord causes the loss of all reflexes for a minimum of about 2 weeks. This is spinal shock. Neurogenic shock describes the cardiovascular instability that occurs with cord transection and is caused by the loss of sympathetic tone and is characterised by hypotension and bradycardia. The return of reflex activity may be due to the sprouting of collaterals from existing neurones, with the formation of additional excitatory endings on interneurones and motor neurones. Autonomic hyperactivity takes a few weeks to develop and is characterised by sweating, pallor and swings in blood pressure. Voluntary control of bladder and bowel function is lost.

Morgan GE, Mikhail MS. *Clinical Anaesthesiology*, 2nd Edn. Appleton and Lange, 1996, Chapter 41

Pinnock CA, Lin ES, Smith T. *Fundamentals of Anaesthesia*, 2nd Edn. Greenwich Medical Media Ltd, 2003, Section 2: Chapter 9

A 141. A. false   **B.** false   **C.** false   **D.** false   **E.** true

In humans, the vast majority of cerebral blood flow is provided by the internal carotid arteries with a relatively small fraction being carried by the vertebral arteries. Cerebral blood flow accounts for approximately 15–20% of cardiac output. There is wide regional variation in CBF and the grey matter may receive 4 times the blood flow of the white matter. CBF is directly proportional to pCO_2 between tensions of 20 and 80 mmHg. The blood flow therefore changes by about 1–2 ml/100 g/min per mmHg change in pCO_2. If intracranial pressure is raised to more than 33 mmHg over a short period, CBF is significantly reduced and the resultant ischaemia stimulates the vasomotor area to increase blood pressure.

Morgan GE, Mikhail MS. *Clinical Anaesthesiology*, 2nd Edn. Appleton and Lange, 1996, Chapter 25

Pinnock CA, Lin ES, Smith T. *Fundamentals of Anaesthesia*, 2nd Edn. Greenwich Medical Media Ltd, 2003, Section 2: Chapter 6

A **142. A.** false **B.** true **C.** false **D.** true **E.** true

Haemoglobin has a molecular weight of 66,700 daltons. Each molecule comprises four haem subunits, each consisting of a polypeptide and a ferrous atom. Adult haemoglobin (HbA1) contains two alpha and two beta chains while foetal haemoglobin (HbF) contains two alpha and two gamma polypeptides. HbF has a lower affinity for binding 2,3-DPG than adult forms of Hb. 2,3-DPG is a highly anionic intermediate of glycolysis and binds to the deoxygenated form of Hb significantly reducing the affinity of Hb for oxygen. Hb-oxygen binding is 'cooperative' meaning that binding O_2 at each site promotes further binding at the remaining sites due to allosteric changes.

Pinnock CA, Lin ES, Smith T. *Fundamentals of Anaesthesia*, 2nd Edn. Greenwich Medical Media Ltd, 2003, Section 2: Chapter 8

A **143. A.** false **B.** true **C.** false **D.** true **E.** true

Sickle cell trait (HbAS) is present when only one chromosome has the sickle gene (i.e. the patient is heterozygous). About 0.5% of black Americans are homozygous and therefore have sickle cell anaemia. Patients with sickle cell trait are generally not anaemic, are asymptomatic and have a normal life span. The Sickledex test detects the presence of HbS by precipitating sickling of the red blood cells on exposure to sodium metabisulphate. However, haemoglobin electrophoresis is necessary to distinguish between the heterozygote and the homozygote.

Morgan GE, Mikhail MS. *Clinical Anaesthesiology*, 2nd Edn. Appleton and Lange, 1996, Chapter 29

Pinnock CA, Lin ES, Smith T. *Fundamentals of Anaesthesia*, 2nd Edn. Greenwich Medical Media Ltd, 2003, Section 1: Chapter 1, Section 2: Chapter 3

A 144. **A.** true   **B.** false   **C.** true   **D.** true   **E.** false

Fibrinogen and globulin levels are increased but the plasma concentration of albumin is reduced. Cardiac output increases by 50%. Heart rate is increased by 25% by the end of the second trimester and stroke volume is increased by 30% at the same time. FRC is decreased by 25–30% at term due to a 25% reduction in expiratory reserve volume and a 15% decrease in residual volume.

Pinnock CA, Lin ES, Smith T. *Fundamentals of Anaesthesia*, 2nd Edn. Greenwich Medical Media Ltd, 2003, Section 2: Chapter 13

A 145. **A.** true   **B.** false   **C.** true   **D.** false   **E.** true

The pulmonary vascular resistance (PVR) is influenced by several factors. Lung volume determines the calibre of the vessels, either being stretched and narrow at high volumes or tortuous at low volumes. PVR is lowest at FRC. Autonomic innervation exerts a weak influence on PVR, with increases in sympathetic tone causing vasoconstriction. During IPPV alveolar pressure may exceed intravascular pressure and therefore increase PVR. Hypoxic pulmonary vasoconstriction is the reason that PVR is high in the foetus and at altitude.

Pinnock CA, Lin ES, Smith T. *Fundamentals of Anaesthesia*, 2nd Edn. Greenwich Medical Media Ltd, 2003, Section 2: Chapter 8

A 146. **A.** false   **B.** false   **C.** false   **D.** true   **E.** false

The nervi erigentes are the efferent parasympathetic nerve supply to the penis. The pain of labour is transmitted via two routes. Firstly from the body and fundus of the uterus via the lower thoracic spinal roots, T10 to L1. Pain impulses from the cervix and birth canal pass via the sacral roots S2 to S4. The pain of the first stage of labour is therefore felt as lower abdominal pain and that of the second stage felt more as pelvic and perineal pain.

Pinnock CA, Lin ES, Smith T. *Fundamentals of Anaesthesia*, 2nd Edn. Greenwich Medical Media Ltd, 2003, Section 1: Chapter 5

A 147. **A.** true   **B.** false   **C.** true   **D.** false   **E.** true

The position of the curve is described by the P50, which is the pO_2 at which Hb is 50% saturated. The normal value is 3.5 kPa. An increased P50 represents a decreased O_2 affinity of Hb. The O_2-myoglobin curve lies to the left of the O_2-Hb curve and is therefore capable of acting as an oxygen store. Cooperative binding describes the effect whereby binding at each O_2 site promotes binding at the remaining sites due to allosteric changes. Stored blood has very little 2,3-DPG and is cold.

Pinnock CA, Lin ES, Smith T. *Fundamentals of Anaesthesia*, 2nd Edn. Greenwich Medical Media Ltd, 2003, Sections 2: Chapters 3, 8

A 148. **A.** true   **B.** true   **C.** false   **D.** false   **E.** false

Pulmonary vascular resistance falls with the first breath. Until then, hypoxic pulmonary vasoconstriction maintains a high PVR. The higher right atrial pressure maintains the foramen ovale patent in utero. Blood flow from the SVC is directed into the right ventricle to preferentially allow blood from the IVC (oxygenated) to enter the left side of the heart and hence the foetal brain. Some blood from the umbilical vein mixes with blood from the portal circulation in the liver and then drains into the IVC via the hepatic vein. Pulmonary capillaries are formed after 24–26 weeks as maturation of the lungs lags behind that of the circulation.

Morgan GE, Mikhail MS. *Clinical Anaesthesiology*, 2nd Edn. Appleton and Lange, 1996, Chapter 42

Pinnock CA, Lin ES, Smith T. *Fundamentals of Anaesthesia*, 2nd Edn. Greenwich Medical Media Ltd, 2003, Section 2: Chapter 14

A. true **B.** true **C.** false **D.** true **E.** true

The relationship between closing capacity and FRC is important because as closing volume encroaches on FRC airway collapse will occur at the end of a normal tidal breath. This will cause problems with gas exchange. This is common in the elderly. The closing volume can be measured by examining nitrogen washout after a single breath of 100% oxygen.

Pinnock CA, Lin ES, Smith T. *Fundamentals of Anaesthesia*, 2nd Edn. Greenwich Medical Media Ltd, 2003, Section 2: Chapter 8

West JB. *Respiratory Physiology – The Essentials*, 5th Edn. Williams & Wilkins, 1995, Chapter 10

A. false **B.** false **C.** true **D.** false **E.** true

A decrease in mean arterial pressure causes cerebral vasodilatation in an attempt to maintain cerebral blood flow. This can raise intracranial pressure due to the increased cerebral blood volume. Low pO_2 vasodilates and high pO_2 vasoconstricts but the effect of oxygen on cerebral vessels is much less marked than that of pCO_2. Jugular venous blood is normally about 65% saturated. Doppler is a crude method of measuring cerebral blood flow but is useful clinically.

Pinnock CA, Lin ES, Smith T. *Fundamentals of Anaesthesia*, 2nd Edn. Greenwich Medical Media Ltd, 2003, Section 2: Chapter 6

Physiology

Answers

A 1.   **A.** true   **B.** true   **C.** true   **D.** true   **E.** false

Tyrosine – DOPA – Dopamine – Noradrenaline – Adrenaline.

Noradrenaline is converted in the adrenal medulla and some neurones to adrenaline, a reaction catalysed by the enzyme phenylethanolamine-N-methyltransferase (PNMT). Adrenaline is a positive inotrope and chronotrope (beta-1) but will reduce total peripheral resistance by dilating blood vessels in skeletal muscle and liver (beta-2). The pulse pressure is therefore widened. Other effects include increased glycogenolysis, increased gluconeogenesis, increased lipolysis and increased metabolic rate.

Pinnock CA, Lin ES, Smith T. *Fundamentals of Anaesthesia*, 2nd Edn. Greenwich Medical Media Ltd, 2003, Section 3

A 2.   **A.** false   **B.** true   **C.** true   **D.** true   **E.** false

Prostaglandins are eicosanoids (related to the C20 acid, eicosanoic acid), naturally occurring substances derived from arachidonic acid. Other groups of eicosanoids include the leukotrienes and thromboxanes.

The main physiologically active prostaglandins are:
- PGD2 – causes vasodilatation and inhibition of platelet aggregation
- PGF2a – luteolysis, uterine contraction and bronchoconstriction
- PgI2 – (prostacyclin) causes vasodilatation and inhibition of platelet aggregation
- PGE2 – there are three subgroups of receptors (EP1-3) causing differing effects:
  - EP1, stimulation of these receptors causes contraction of bronchial and gastrointestinal smooth muscle.
  - EP2, bronchodilatation, vasodilatation and GIT smooth muscle relaxation.

— EP3, GIT smooth muscle contraction, inhibition of gastric acid secretion but increased gastric mucus secretion, uterine contraction, inhibition of lipolysis and autonomic neurotransmitter release.

There is a high concentration of a prostaglandin specific enzyme in the lung.

PGD2 is stored in mast cells.

Rang HP, Dale MM, Ritter JM. *Pharmacology*, 4th Edn. Churchill Livingstone, 1999, Chapter 12

A 3. **A.** false **B.** false **C.** false **D.** false **E.** true

Alpha-1 stimulation causes vasoconstriction, intestinal smooth muscle relaxation, increased saliva secretion and hepatic glycogenolysis. Chronotropic and inotropic effects are via beta-receptors.

Pinnock CA, Lin ES, Smith T. *Fundamentals of Anaesthesia*, 2nd Edn. Greenwich Medical Media Ltd, 2003, Section 3: Chapter 11

A 4. **A.** true **B.** true **C.** false **D.** true **E.** true

Ringer lactate contains 2 mmol/l of calcium.

Pinnock CA, Lin ES, Smith T. *Fundamentals of Anaesthesia*, 2nd Edn. Greenwich Medical Media Ltd, 2003, Section 3: Chapter 16

A 5. **A.** true **B.** true **C.** false **D.** true **E.** true

Digoxin stimulates vagal activity slowing conduction and prolonging the refractory period in the AV node and bundle. It has a narrow therapeutic window and is therefore liable to complications following accidental or deliberate overdose. Clinical features of toxicity include non-specific symptoms such as nausea, vomiting, anorexia, abdominal pain, visual disturbances and headache. Cardiac toxicity can be associated with bradycardia, AV block, supraventricular arrhythmias and ventricular arrhythmias. Management will be guided by the arrhythmia but may include atropine/pacing for bradycardia, phenytoin/lidocaine for ventricular arrhythmias as well as correction of electrolytes (especially potassium) and the use of digoxin-specific antibody fragments (Fab).

Hinds CJ, Watson D. *Intensive Care – A Concise Textbook*. WB Saunders, 1995

A **6.** **A.** true **B.** false **C.** true **D.** true **E.** true

Side effects of steroid therapy may be divided into:
1. Mineralocorticoid – sodium retention, potassium loss, water retention, renal calcium loss, hypertension, and;
2. Glucocorticoid – muscle wasting, fat deposition, liver glycogen deposition, thin friable skin, poor wound healing, reduced immunity, cataracts, raised intraocular pressure, osteoporosis and hyperglycaemia.

Pinnock CA, Lin ES, Smith T. *Fundamentals of Anaesthesia*, 2nd Edn. Greenwich Medical Media Ltd, 2003, Section 3: Chapter 14

A **7.** **A.** true **B.** true **C.** true **D.** false **E.** true

The rate of uptake of anaesthetic agents from inspired gas to the blood is determined during the pulmonary phase by the following factors – inhaled concentration, alveolar minute ventilation, diffusion, blood/gas partition coefficient, partial pressure of agent in the pulmonary artery, pulmonary blood flow (cardiac output), ventilation/perfusion distribution, concentration effect and the second gas effect.

Pinnock CA, Lin ES, Smith T. *Fundamentals of Anaesthesia*, 2nd Edn. Greenwich Medical Media Ltd, 2003, Section 3: Chapter 5

A **8.** **A.** false **B.** false **C.** false **D.** true **E.** false

Acetylcholinesterase is present on the junctional clefts of the postsynaptic membrane (also some presynaptical) while pseudocholinesterase is found in plasma. Pilocarpine is a naturally occurring cholinomimetic substance, used as a miotic agent. Dibucaine is a local anaesthetic agent used to determine variations in plasma cholinesterase activity (it selective inhibits the normal enzyme).

Pinnock CA, Lin ES, Smith T. *Fundamentals of Anaesthesia*, 2nd Edn. Greenwich Medical Media Ltd, 2003, Section 3: Chapter 8

Rang HP, Dale MM, Ritter JM. *Pharmacology*, 4th Edn. Churchill Livingstone, 1999

A **9.** **A.** true **B.** false **C.** false **D.** true **E.** true

The mode of action of paracetamol is still (amazingly) ill understood. It is known to inhibit prostaglandin synthesis in the CNS which accounts for its antipyretic activity. Only <5% is protein-bound and the oral bioavailability is 70–90%. It is metabolised predominantly in the liver to form glucuronide, sulphate and cystine conjugates.

Pinnock CA, Lin ES, Smith T. *Fundamentals of Anaesthesia*, 2nd Edn. Greenwich Medical Media Ltd, 2003, Section 3: Chapter 7

A 10. **A.** false **B.** true **C.** true **D.** true **E.** false

The boiling point of ether is 35°C and that of trichloroethylene is 87°C.

Pinnock CA, Lin ES, Smith T. *Fundamentals of Anaesthesia*, 2nd Edn. Greenwich Medical Media Ltd, 2003, Section 3: Chapter 5

A 11. **A.** true **B.** true **C.** true **D.** true **E.** true

Idiosyncratic side effects include acne, gum hyperplasia, coarsened facies, megaloblastic anaemia and other blood dyscrasias, osteomalacia, systemic lupus erythematosus (SLE), hepatotoxicity and allergic phenomena. There are also concentration dependent side effects including nausea and vomiting, drowsiness, behavioural disturbance, tremor, ataxia, nystagmus, peripheral neuropathy and cerebellar damage.

Sasada M, Smith S. *Drugs in Anaesthesia and Intensive Care*, 2nd Edn. Oxford University Press, 1997, p 298

A 12. **A.** true **B.** true **C.** false **D.** false **E.** false

Morphine is predominantly metabolised in the liver, undergoing phase 1 reaction (oxidative N dealkylation) and phase 2 reaction (conjugation with glucuronide).

Conjugation occurs at the 3- and 6-OH groups to form morphine-3-glucuronide and morphine-6-glucuronide. The glucuronides are hydrolysed in the GIT and most of the morphine is reabsorbed.

Pinnock CA, Lin ES, Smith T. *Fundamentals of Anaesthesia*, 2nd Edn. Greenwich Medical Media Ltd, 2003, Section 3, p 625

A 13. **A.** false **B.** false **C.** false **D.** false **E.** true

Monoamine oxidase (MAO) exists in two similar molecular forms which have relative substrate preferences. MAO-A has a preference for 5-HT and MAO-B for phenylethylamine while both act on noradrenaline and dopamine. Monoamine oxidase inhibitors (MAOI) cause a sustained increase in 5-HT, noradrenaline and dopamine. Most are irreversible and relatively non-selective.

Side effects include postural hypotension (sympathetic block), excessive CNS stimulation (tremors, excitement, insomnia, convulsions), weight gain, and atropine-like side effects.

Co-administration of indirectly acting sympathomimetic amines can result in severe hypertension. Tyramine (from cheese, red wine, Marmite) is a monoamine normally metabolised by MAO in the gut wall and liver and can also lead to severe hypertension if ingested by someone taking MAOIs. There is a specific reaction with pethidine leading to hyperpyrexia, hypertension and coma, the cause of which is poorly defined.

Pinnock CA, Lin ES, Smith T. *Fundamentals of Anaesthesia*, 2nd Edn. Greenwich Medical Media Ltd, 2003, Section 3, p 676

Rang HP, Dale MM, Ritter JM. *Pharmacology*, 4th Edn. Churchill Livingstone, 1999, p 559

A 14. A. true **B.** true **C.** false **D.** false **E.** true

Isoflurane is a halogenated methyl ether and a structural isomer of enflurane. It is a respiratory depressant by reducing tidal volume. Only 0.2% is metabolised in the liver by oxidation and dehalogenation. It causes a drop in systemic vascular resistance with a compensatory tachycardia. Enflurane is epileptogenic.

Pinnock CA, Lin ES, Smith T. *Fundamentals of Anaesthesia*, 2nd Edn. Greenwich Medical Media Ltd, 2003, Section 3, p 597

Sasada M, Smith S. *Drugs in Anaesthesia and Intensive Care*, 2nd Edn. Oxford University Press, 1997, p 208

A 15. A. true **B.** false **C.** false **D.** true **E.** true

Metabolism of bupivacaine (an amide local anaesthetic agent) occurs in the liver by N-dealkylation while 16% is excreted unchanged in the urine. The pKa of bupivacaine is 8.1 so it is 50% ionised at this pH. Central nervous system side effects occur before cardiovascular side effects but once myocardial depression happens, it is slow to reverse (it binds to myocardial proteins).

Sasada M, Smith S. *Drugs in Anaesthesia and Intensive Care*, 2nd Edn. Oxford University Press, 1997, p 52

A **16.** **A.** false **B.** true **C.** false **D.** false **E.** false

Ritodrine is a beta-2 agonist which relaxes uterine smooth muscle and is used to delay delivery in premature labour. Side effects include nausea and vomiting, sweating, tremor, hypokalaemia, tachycardia, hypotension, pulmonary oedema and arrhythmias.

British National Formulary. Published by the British Medical Association & The Royal Pharmaceutical Society of Great Britain

A **17.** **A.** true **B.** false **C.** true **D.** false **E.** false

Propofol has anticonvulsant properties and there is no evidence that the drug produces epileptiform activity in non-epileptic patients. It is presented as an oil/water emulsion and causes pain on injection in up to 30% of cases. It is an alkyl phenol unlike etomidate which is an imidazole. 98% is protein bound.

Pinnock CA, Lin ES, Smith T. *Fundamentals of Anaesthesia*, 2nd Edn. Greenwich Medical Media Ltd, 2003, Section 3, p 610

Sasada M, Smith S. *Drugs in Anaesthesia and Intensive Care*, 2nd Edn. Oxford University Press, 1997, p 314

A **18.** **A.** true **B.** false **C.** false **D.** true **E.** false

Ondansetron is a selective 5-HT-3 antagonist acting both centrally and peripherally (small intestine). Apomorphine is a dopaminergic drug used in Parkinsonism. Patients are established on domperidone for at least 2 days before starting apomorphine.

Sasada M, Smith S. *Drugs in Anaesthesia and Intensive Care*, 2nd Edn. Oxford University Press, 1997

A **19.** **A.** true **B.** false **C.** true **D.** false **E.** true

Arachidonic acid is derived from phospholipid and has many metabolites depending on the enzyme involved. The action of cyclo-oxygenase can give rise to prostaglandins, prostacyclin and thromboxane while the action of 5-lipoxygenase can lead to the formation of the leukotrienes.

Bradykinin is a vasoactive nonapeptide clipped out of kininogen by a proteolytic enzyme, kallikrein.

Angiotensin 1 is a decapeptide cleaved off angiotensinogen by the action of renin.

Rang HP, Dale MM, Ritter JM. *Pharmacology*, 4th Edn. Churchill Livingstone, 1999

A **20.** **A.** false **B.** false **C.** false **D.** true **E.** false

Temazepam is a 1,4-benzodiazepine which is available in tablet and elixir form only. It acts as an agonist at a subtype of the benzodiazepine receptor (BDZ1-3) which is attached to the GABA receptor complex on the postsynaptic membrane.
The terminal half-life of temazepam is 4–10 h while that of midazolam is 1–3 h.

Pinnock CA, Lin ES, Smith T. *Fundamentals of Anaesthesia*, 2nd Edn. Greenwich Medical Media Ltd, 2003, Section 3, p 611

A **21.** **A.** false **B.** true **C.** false **D.** true **E.** false

Isoflurane causes a decrease in tidal volume with either a normal or slightly raised respiratory rate – the result is a slight rise in $PaCO_2$. It does cause catecholamine sensitisation but less than that seen with halothane or enflurane. Isoflurane is pungent and causes some respiratory irritation, making inhalational induction difficult. It has a MAC value of 1.15 (halothane is 0.75)

Pinnock CA, Lin ES, Smith T. *Fundamentals of Anaesthesia*, 2nd Edn. Greenwich Medical Media Ltd, 2003, Section 3, p 597

A **22.** **A.** false **B.** true **C.** false **D.** false **E.** true

Morphine is well absorbed but undergoes extensive first-pass metabolism. Neomycin is poorly absorbed and has been used for bowel sterilisation.

A **23.** **A.** false **B.** true **C.** true **D.** false **E.** true

Opioid receptors are all G-protein coupled receptors and exist in the CNS and peripheral sites such as the gastrointestinal tract. There are three types of opioid receptors, distinguished by their prototype agonists – OP1 (delta), OP2 (kappa) and OP3 (mu). Stimulation of μ-receptors leads to analgesia, euphoria and some degree of axniolysis. Substance P is a polypeptide and in conjunction with glutamine may be involved in 'wind up' by its action on NMDA receptors. The intrathecal administration of opioids requires the dose to be substantially reduced to produce the same analgesia.

Pinnock CA, Lin ES, Smith T. *Fundamentals of Anaesthesia*, 2nd Edn. Greenwich Medical Media Ltd, 2003, Section 3, p 621

A 24. A. false **B.** false **C.** true **D.** true **E.** true

The aminoglycosides include gentamicin, neomycin, netilmicin, streptomycin, tobramycin and amikacin. Most side effects are dose-related and the important ones are ototoxicity and nephrotoxicity. They also impair neuromuscular transmission. The action of non-depolarising muscle relaxants is prolonged by inhibiting presynaptic acetylcholine release and by stabilisation of the postsynaptic membrane at the neuromuscular junction.

Pinnock CA, Lin ES, Smith T. *Fundamentals of Anaesthesia*, 2nd Edn. Greenwich Medical Media Ltd, 2003, Section 3: Chapter 18

Sasada M, Smith S. *Drugs in Anaesthesia and Intensive Care*, 2nd Edn. Oxford University Press, 1997

A 25. A. false **B.** true **C.** true **D.** false **E.** false

Suxamethonium is hydrolysed by plasma cholinesterase to succinylomonocholine (which has some weak activity) and choline. Succinylomonocholine is further hydrolysed to succinic acid and choline. Plasma cholinesterase activity may be reduced in certain conditions (pregnancy, liver disease, cardiac and renal failure, burns) and by certain drugs (ecothiopate, tacrine, lidocaine, procaine, lithium, magnesium, ketamine, pancuronium, OCP and cytotoxic agents).

Pinnock CA, Lin ES, Smith T. *Fundamentals of Anaesthesia*, 2nd Edn. Greenwich Medical Media Ltd, 2003, Section 3

Sasada M, Smith S. *Drugs in Anaesthesia and Intensive Care*, 2nd Edn. Oxford University Press, 1997

A 26. A. false **B.** true **C.** false **D.** true **E.** true

Propanolol (a non-selective beta-blocker with no intrinsic sympathomimetic activity) is used in the treatment of a number of areas including hypertension, angina, phaeochromocytoma, essential tremor, anxiety, thyrotoxicosis and migraine. It reduces plasma renin activity and suppresses aldosterone release. As a beta-2 antagonist, it can lead to bronchoconstriction.

Sasada M, Smith S. *Drugs in Anaesthesia and Intensive Care*, 2nd Edn. Oxford University Press, 1997

A 27. A. false **B.** true **C.** false **D.** true **E.** true

Dopamine antagonists (phenothiazines, butyrophenones, metoclopramide, domperidone) are ineffective in motion sickness where antimuscarinics or antihistamines are indicated. Interference of autonomic regulation by the hypothalamus can lead to severe hypotension (as well as alpha-adrenoceptor blockade). Neuroleptanalgesia was introduced in 1959 and commonly used a butyrophenone in conjunction with a potent opioid.

Calvey TN, Williams NE. *Principles and Practice of Pharmacology for Anaesthesia*, 4th Edn. Blackwell Science, 2001

A 28. A. false **B.** false **C.** false **D.** false **E.** true

Gentamicin is not significantly absorbed orally. Propanolol is 90% absorbed but undergoes extensive first-pass metabolism giving a bioavailability of 30–35%. Morphine similarly is well absorbed and metabolised with a bioavailability of 15–50%. The bioavailability of atenolol is 50%. Unusually for an opioid, methadone has a high oral bioavailability.

Calvey TN, Williams NE. *Principles and Practice of Pharmacology for Anaesthesia*, 4th Edn. Blackwell Science, 2001

Pinnock CA, Lin ES, Smith T. *Fundamentals of Anaesthesia*, 2nd Edn. Greenwich Medical Media Ltd, 2003, Section 3

A 29. A. true **B.** true **C.** true **D.** false **E.** true

Allopurinol inhibits xanthine oxidase. Physostigmine is a naturally occurring anticholinesterase drug. Indomethacin reduces prostaglandin production by inhibiting cyclo-oxygenase. Enoxomone is a selective phosphodiesterase inhibitor. Meptazinol is an opioid agonist.

Pinnock CA, Lin ES, Smith T. *Fundamentals of Anaesthesia*, 2nd Edn. Greenwich Medical Media Ltd, 2003, Section 3

A **30.** **A.** true   **B.** false   **C.** true   **D.** false   **E.** false

Morphine delays gastric emptying while metoclopramide increases gastrointestinal motility and gastric emptying. Ranitidine increases lower oesophageal tone but has no effect on gastric emptying. Sucralfate is used for cytoprotection of the upper GIT but does not affect gastric emptying.

Sasada M, Smith S. *Drugs in Anaesthesia and Intensive Care*, 2nd Edn. Oxford University Press, 1997

A **31.** **A.** false   **B.** true   **C.** false   **D.** true   **E.** true

Nalorphine and pentazocine are mixed agonist-antagonists at opioid receptors. Ketocyclazocine is the prototype agonist for the OP2 (kappa) opioid receptor. Clonidine is an alpha-2 agonist while diazepam acts at benzodiazepine/GABA receptors.

Pinnock CA, Lin ES, Smith T. *Fundamentals of Anaesthesia*, 2nd Edn. Greenwich Medical Media Ltd, 2003

Rang HP, Dale MM, Ritter JM. *Pharmacology*, 4th Edn. Churchill Livingstone, 1999

A **32.** **A.** false   **B.** false   **C.** false   **D.** true   **E.** true

Diacetyl morphine (diamorphine) is a prodrug and acts via its active derivatives (morphine and 6-0-acetylmorphine) which are μ-opioid receptor agonists. Naloxone and naltrexone are opioid antagonists – naltrexone has a much longer duration of action. Pentazocine is a mixed agonist-antagonist while buprenorphine is a partial agonist at μ-receptors.

Rang HP, Dale MM, Ritter JM. *Pharmacology*, 4th Edn. Churchill Livingstone, 1999

Sasada M, Smith S. *Drugs in Anaesthesia and Intensive Care*, 2nd Edn. Oxford University Press, 1997

A **33.** **A.** false   **B.** false   **C.** false   **D.** true   **E.** true

Enflurane is a halogenated ether with a MAC value of 1.68 (halothane 0.75). Its boiling point is 56.5°C, that of halothane is 50.2°C. All the volatile agents potentiate neuromuscular blockade. 2.4% of enflurane is metabolised producing inorganic fluoride ions.

Pinnock CA, Lin ES, Smith T. *Fundamentals of Anaesthesia*, 2nd Edn. Greenwich Medical Media Ltd, 2003, Section 3: Chapter 5

A 34. A. false **B.** true **C.** false **D.** false **E.** true

Atropine is the ester of tropic acid and tropine (hyoscine is the ester of tropic acid and scopine). It is presented as a racemic mixture of D- and l-isomers (l-form is active). Inhibition of sweating may lead to hyperpyrexia in children. It increases physiological dead space and like hyoscine crosses the blood-brain barrier.

Sasada M, Smith S. *Drugs in Anaesthesia and Intensive Care*, 2nd Edn. Oxford University Press, 1997

A 35. A. true **B.** false **C.** false **D.** true **E.** true

As a sympathomimetic phenylephrine causes mydriasis, neostigmine leads to miosis. Glycopyrrolate does not cross the blood-brain barrier and has no effect on pupil size or accommodation. Pancuronium (a bis-quaternary aminosteroid) does not cross the blood-brain barrier. Trimetaphan is a competitive ganglion blocker used to produce hypotension and causes mydriasis.

Sasada M, Smith S. *Drugs in Anaesthesia and Intensive Care*, 2nd Edn. Oxford University Press, 1997

A 36. A. true **B.** false **C.** true **D.** false **E.** false

In common with other benzodiazepines, diazepam has anticonvulsant properties. It is a 1,4-benzodiazepine (no imidazole ring unlike midazolam) which is insoluble in water. It is metabolised in the liver and its main metabolite is desmethyldiazepam but oxazepam is also formed. Its elimination half-life is 20–40 h.

Pinnock CA, Lin ES, Smith T. *Fundamentals of Anaesthesia*, 2nd Edn. Greenwich Medical Media Ltd, 2003, Section 3: Chapter 10

Pharmacology

Answers

A 37. A. true **B.** false **C.** true **D.** false **E.** false

Dantrolene (1–10 mg/kg i.v.) is used in the treatment of malignant hyperthermia. It inhibits muscle contraction by preventing calcium release from the sarcoplasmic reticulum. It is not a opiate antagonist although it may have some GABA-related effects. It has minimal respiratory effects.

Sasada M, Smith S. *Drugs in Anaesthesia and Intensive Care*, 2nd Edn. Oxford University Press, 1997

A 38. A. true **B.** true **C.** false **D.** true **E.** false

Atracurium is a benzyl-isoquinolinium ester used as a competitive neuromuscular blocker. It undergoes both Hoffmann elimination (to laudanosine and a quaternary monoacrylate) and ester hydrolysis. The metabolites are inactive. Atracurium should be stored in the fridge at 2–8°C.

Pinnock CA, Lin ES, Smith T. *Fundamentals of Anaesthesia*, 2nd Edn. Greenwich Medical Media Ltd, 2003, Section 3: Chapter 8

A 39. A. false **B.** true **C.** true **D.** false **E.** true

Neostigmine, a quaternary amine, is highly ionised and does not cross the blood-brain barrier. Physostigmine has tertiary groups and does therefore cross.

Pinnock CA, Lin ES, Smith T. *Fundamentals of Anaesthesia*, 2nd Edn. Greenwich Medical Media Ltd, 2003, Section 3

A 40. A. true **B.** false **C.** false **D.** false **E.** false

Midazolam has a imidazole ring which is open at pH 3 making it water soluble. The ring closes above pH 4 and the drug is then lipid soluble. Atracurium is stored in acid conditions and is degraded at more physiological pH. Both methohexitone and thiopentone change their degree of ionisation (rather than structural changes) with changes in pH.

Pinnock CA, Lin ES, Smith T. *Fundamentals of Anaesthesia*, 2nd Edn. Greenwich Medical Media Ltd, 2003, Section 3

A 41. A. true **B.** true **C.** true **D.** true **E.** false

Reduced plasma cholinesterase activity may be due to a deficiency of the molecules or an abnormality of the enzyme. Causes of plasma cholinesterase deficiency are numerous and include pregnancy, hypoproteinaemia, liver disease, carcinomatosis and many drugs (e.g. ketamine, pancuronium, propanolol, ecothiopate eye drops, oral contraceptives and amethocaine).

Pinnock CA, Lin ES, Smith T. *Fundamentals of Anaesthesia*, 2nd Edn. Greenwich Medical Media Ltd, 2003, Section 3

A **42.** **A.** true **B.** true **C.** false **D.** true **E.** true

Orally administered magnesium sulphate acts as an osmotic diuretic.

Pinnock CA, Lin ES, Smith T. *Fundamentals of Anaesthesia*, 2nd Edn. Greenwich Medical Media Ltd, 2003, Section 3: Chapter 15

A **43.** **A.** true **B.** false **C.** true **D.** true **E.** false

The synthesis of catecholamines runs from phenylalanine – tyrosine – DOPA – dopamine – norepinephrine – epinephrine. Methionine is used in paracetamol overdose to increase glutathione formation in the liver. Isoprenaline is a synthetic catecholamine.

Pinnock CA, Lin ES, Smith T. *Fundamentals of Anaesthesia*, 2nd Edn. Greenwich Medical Media Ltd, 2003, Section 3: Chapter 11

A **44.** **A.** true **B.** false **C.** true **D.** false **E.** false

Osmotic diuretics (e.g. mannitol) are used in the treatment of raised intracranial pressure and raised intraocular pressure as well as for their diuretic and antioxidant effects. Side effects include hypokalaemia, hyponatraemia and increased plasma osmolality.

Sasada M, Smith S. *Drugs in Anaesthesia and Intensive Care*, 2nd Edn. Oxford University Press, 1997

A **45.** **A.** false **B.** true **C.** false **D.** false **E.** true

Thiazide diuretics work on the luminal membrane pump of the distal convoluted tubule by inhibiting active sodium and chloride reabsorption. Magnesium excretion is increased but calcium and uric acid excretion are reduced. They are best avoided in diabetics owing to their ability to cause hyperglycaemia.

Pinnock CA, Lin ES, Smith T. *Fundamentals of Anaesthesia*, 2nd Edn. Greenwich Medical Media Ltd, 2003, Section 3: Chapter 12

A 46. **A.** true   **B.** true   **C.** true   **D.** true   **E.** false

Ketamine is a phencyclidine derivative presented as a racemic mixture. It increases heart rate, blood pressure and catecholamine levels by a generalised increase in CNS activity. Muscle tone is increased and it may lead to generalised muscle rigidity. Problems with ketamine include unpleasant dreams, hallucinations, emergence delirium and pain on injection. It increases uterine tone.

Pinnock CA, Lin ES, Smith T. *Fundamentals of Anaesthesia*, 2nd Edn. Greenwich Medical Media Ltd, 2003, Section 3: Chapter 6

A 47. **A.** true   **B.** false   **C.** false   **D.** true   **E.** true

Competitive neuromuscular blockade is prolonged in the presence of hypokalaemia, hypocalcaemia, hypermagnesaemia, hypoproteinaemia, dehydration, acidosis and hypercapnia. Some drugs also enhance the block (e.g. volatile agents, suxamethonium, calcium antagonists, protamine, fentanyl, prtamine, alpha- and beta-antagonists, metronidazole and aminoglycosides).

Sasada M, Smith S. *Drugs in Anaesthesia and Intensive Care*, 2nd Edn. Oxford University Press, 1997

A 48. **A.** true   **B.** true   **C.** true   **D.** false   **E.** false

There is an increase in sympathetic tone following the administration of ketamine with a resultant increase in heart rate, blood pressure and cardiac output. Nitrous oxide has mild myocardial depressant effects but increases sympathetic activity (central effect) with little overall effect on haemodynamic parameters.

Calvey TN, Williams NE. *Principles and Practice of Pharmacology for Anaesthesia*, 4th Edn. Blackwell Science, 2001

Sasada M, Smith S. *Drugs in Anaesthesia and Intensive Care*, 2nd Edn. Oxford University Press, 1997

A 49. **A.** true   **B.** true   **C.** false   **D.** true   **E.** false

Methaemoglobinaemia occurs when there is increased Fe^{3+} in haemoglobin and it is an ineffective oxygen carrier. It can be congenital or acquired. Acquired methaemoglobinaemia is associated with certain drugs, e.g. prilocaine, chlorate, quinones, nitrates and sulphonamides. The treatment is with methylene blue 1–2 mg/kg.

Yentis S, Hirsch N, Smith G. *Anaesthesia A to Z*. Butterworth-Heinemann, 1995

A 50. A. true **B.** false **C.** true **D.** false **E.** true

Verapamil, a synthetic papaverine derivative, causes competitive blockade of slow calcium channels reducing calcium influx into vascular smooth muscle and myocardial cells. The effect in the heart is to reduce automaticity and conduction velocity with an increase in the refractory period. A-V conduction is slowed. Cardiac contractility is reduced. Similarly coronary and systemic arteries dilate so afterload is reduced.

Pinnock CA, Lin ES, Smith T. *Fundamentals of Anaesthesia*, 2nd Edn. Greenwich Medical Media Ltd, 2003, Section 3: Chapter 12

Sasada M, Smith S. *Drugs in Anaesthesia and Intensive Care*, 2nd Edn. Oxford University Press, 1997

A 51. A. true **B.** false **C.** false **D.** true **E.** true

Digoxin is a cardiac glycoside with a low therapeutic index (therapeutic range 1–2 ng/ml). Digoxin toxicity can lead to most forms of dysrhythmia but junctional bradycardia and ventricular bigemini are common. Hypokalaemia, hypernatraemia, hypercalcaemia and hypomagnesaemia increase the likelihood of toxicity. Electrolyte disturbances should be corrected during treatment, phentoin and lidocaine have been used for ventricular arrhythmias and digoxin-specific antibody fragments are used in severe toxicity. Beta-blockers should be avoided.

Hinds CJ, Watson D. *Intensive Care – A Concise Textbook*. WB Saunders, 1995

Sasada M, Smith S. *Drugs in Anaesthesia and Intensive Care*, 2nd Edn. Oxford University Press, 1997

A 52. A. false **B.** false **C.** false **D.** true **E.** true

Phenytoin can cause hypotension and cardiovascular collapse on injection. Glucagon is a marked positive iontrope and a positive chronotrope to a lesser degree.

Pinnock CA, Lin ES, Smith T. *Fundamentals of Anaesthesia*, 2nd Edn. Greenwich Medical Media Ltd, 2003, Section 3

A **53.** **A.** false **B.** false **C.** true **D.** true **E.** true

Isoprenaline, a synthetic catecholamine, has mainly beta-agonist effects increasing cardiac output (positive inotrope/chronotrope) and reducing peripheral vascular resistance (beta-2 effect). It can cause hyperglycaemia and increase plasma free fatty acids.

Sasada M, Smith S. *Drugs in Anaesthesia and Intensive Care*, 2nd Edn. Oxford University Press, 1997

A **54.** **A.** true **B.** false **C.** true **D.** true **E.** false

Lidocaine has Class 1b antiarrhythmic actions, blocking sodium channels and preventing depolarisation of the cell membrane. It is used for the treatment of ventricular dysrhythmias post-MI. It decreases the rate of phase IV depolarisation, duration of action potential, effective refractory period and conduction velocity.

Pinnock CA, Lin ES, Smith T. *Fundamentals of Anaesthesia*, 2nd Edn. Greenwich Medical Media Ltd, 2003

Sasada M, Smith S. *Drugs in Anaesthesia and Intensive Care*, 2nd Edn. Oxford University Press, 1997

A **55.** **A.** false **B.** true **C.** true **D.** true **E.** false

Atropine causes a reduction in ADH secretion. In low doses there may be a transient bradycardia preceding the normal tachycardia. It can cause cycloplegia, mydriasis and an increase in intraocular pressure. Urinary tract tone is reduced. Atropine has marked antimuscarinic activity but minimal antinicotinic activity.

Sasada M, Smith S. *Drugs in Anaesthesia and Intensive Care*, 2nd Edn. Oxford University Press, 1997

A **56.** **A.** false **B.** false **C.** false **D.** true **E.** false

Isoprenaline and ritodrine both have beta-2 agonist activity and are therefore bronchodilators. Atropine produces bronchodilation and an increase in physiological dead space. Neostigmine can lead to an increase in bronchial secretions and bronchoconstriction.

Pinnock CA, Lin ES, Smith T. *Fundamentals of Anaesthesia*, 2nd Edn. Greenwich Medical Media Ltd, 2003, Section 3

A 57. **A.** false **B.** true **C.** true **D.** true **E.** false

The lipid solubility of these drugs will predict their pharmacokinetic behaviour (e.g. absorption, bioavailability, elimination half-life and transfer across the blood-brain barrier). All the beta-blockers will have some degree of beta-1 and beta-2 activity – metoprolol is relatively selective for beta-2 adrenoceptors and therefore has some degree of cardioselectivity. The intrinsic sympathetic activity of the drugs does not relate to their clinical usefulness.

Calvey TN, Williams NE. *Principles and Practice of Pharmacology for Anaesthesia*, 4th Edn. Blackwell Science, 2001

A 58. **A.** false **B.** true **C.** false **D.** false **E.** false

Physostigmine and atropine are involved mainly in muscarinic effects. Curare is a competitive antagonist of acetylcholine at nicotinic (N2) receptors. Scopolamine is hyscine. Ergotamine is an ergot alkaloid acting at 5-HT1 receptors and used in the treatment of migraine.

Rang HP, Dale MM, Ritter JM. *Pharmacology*, 4th Edn. Churchill Livingstone, 1999

A 59. **A.** true **B.** true **C.** false **D.** false **E.** false

Sodium nitroprusside is used to produce vasodilation and hypotension. It dilates initially the venous system and then arterioles as the dose increases. There is a compensatory tachycardia and cardiac output is maintained. Myocardial contractility is unaltered. SNP metabolism varies with the concentration present. At higher concentrations it undergoes hydrolysis in red blood cells to yield five cyanide ions. One combines with haemoglobin to form methaemoglobin while the other four react with thiosulphate to form thiocyanate. Thiocyanate is excreted unchanged in the urine.

Pinnock CA, Lin ES, Smith T. *Fundamentals of Anaesthesia*, 2nd Edn. Greenwich Medical Media Ltd, 2003, Section 3: Chapter 12

Sasada M, Smith S. *Drugs in Anaesthesia and Intensive Care*, 2nd Edn. Oxford University Press, 1997

A **60.** **A.** true **B.** true **C.** true **D.** true **E.** false

Nifedipine, a dihydropyridine derivative, is a competitive antagonist at slow calcium channels leading to relaxation of arterial smooth muscle in both coronary and peripheral circulations. Like verapamil it is well absorbed orally but verapamil undergoes much more extensive first-pass metabolism.

Sasada M, Smith S. *Drugs in Anaesthesia and Intensive Care*, 2nd Edn. Oxford University Press, 1997

A **61.** **A.** false **B.** true **C.** false **D.** true **E.** true

Atropine is an ester of tropic acid and tropine while hyoscine is an ester of tropic acid and scopine. It does increase physiological dead space and in children leads to decreased sweating and can cause hyperpyrexia. In small doses it may result in bradycardia.

Sasada M, Smith S. *Drugs in Anaesthesia and Intensive Care*, 2nd Edn. Oxford University Press, 1997

A **62.** **A.** true **B.** true **C.** true **D.** true **E.** false

Prazosin is an alpha-1 antagonist causing vascular dilation. Metolazone, like other thiazide diuretics, causes peripheral vasodilation the mechanism of which has not been fully explained.

Calvey TN, Williams NE. *Principles and Practice of Pharmacology for Anaesthesia*, 4th Edn. Blackwell Science, 2001

A **63.** **A.** true **B.** true **C.** true **D.** false **E.** false

Halothane is 1-bromo-1-chloro-2,2,2-trifluoroethane and therefore contains three fluoride atoms. The SVP of halothane is 32.5 kPa at 20°C, its molecular weight is 196.4 daltons, its boiling point 50.2°C and its MAC value 0.75. Vapourisers are calibrated for specific agents and in addition, halothane contains 0.01% thymol which can build-up in the vapouriser chamber.

Pinnock CA, Lin ES, Smith T. *Fundamentals of Anaesthesia*, 2nd Edn. Greenwich Medical Media Ltd, 2003, Section 3: Chapter 5

A **64.** **A.** true **B.** false **C.** true **D.** false **E.** false

Desflurane, enflurane and isoflurane are methyl ethyl ethers. The tachycardia sometimes associated with isoflurane is secondary to hypotension and the drug does not affect AV nodal conduction. The volatiles reduce calcium ion release from the sarcoplasmic reticulum and decrease calcium flux into cardiac cells. Thus the negative inotropic effects of nifedipine are additive in the presence of volatile agents. Isoflurane is a coronary vasodilator and has been implicated in the coronary steal syndrome whereby blood is diverted from stenosed, diseased vessels. Cerebral vasodilation leads to a marginal increase in cerebral blood flow.

Pinnock CA, Lin ES, Smith T. *Fundamentals of Anaesthesia*, 2nd Edn. Greenwich Medical Media Ltd, 2003, Section 3: Chapter 5

Sasada M, Smith S. *Drugs in Anaesthesia and Intensive Care*, 2nd Edn. Oxford University Press, 1997

A **65.** **A.** false **B.** true **C.** true **D.** false **E.** false

Heparin is a mixture of mucopolysaccharides with molecular weights ranging from 3,000–40,000 daltons. It is acidic and has a strong electronegative charge. It binds to and activates antithrombin III, increasing the APTT, thrombin time and activated clotting time but does not affect the bleeding time. It is reversed by protamine, a basic cationic protein which neutralises heparin. Its half-life is 40–120 min. Side effects include thrombocytopaenia, hyperkalaemia and osteoporosis.

Pinnock CA, Lin ES, Smith T. *Fundamentals of Anaesthesia*, 2nd Edn. Greenwich Medical Media Ltd, 2003, Section 3: Chapter 17

A **66.** **A.** true **B.** true **C.** false **D.** false **E.** false

The incidence of unpleasant side effects associated with ketamine can be reduced by premedication with benzodiazepines or butyrophenones (e.g. droperidol). They are less frequent in the young and elderly and after longer procedures. Both isomers of ketamine undergo metabolism in the liver to form norketamine which has less potency than ketamine.

Pinnock CA, Lin ES, Smith T. *Fundamentals of Anaesthesia*, 2nd Edn. Greenwich Medical Media Ltd, 2003, Section 3: Chapter 6

A 67. **A.** false **B.** false **C.** false **D.** false **E.** false

Prilocaine, an amide local anaesthetic, is 55% protein bound mainly to alpha-1 acid glycoprotein. EMLA cream is a eutectic (50:50) mixture of 2.5% prilocaine and 2.5% lidocaine. The ester local anaesthetics are metabolised by plasma cholinesterases while the amides are metabolised in the liver. Prilocaine metabolism can lead to the build-up of o-toluidine which can lead to the development of methaemoglobinaemia. Prilocaine is less toxic than lidocaine.

Pinnock CA, Lin ES, Smith T. *Fundamentals of Anaesthesia*, 2nd Edn. Greenwich Medical Media Ltd, 2003, Section 3: Chapter 9

Sasada M, Smith S. *Drugs in Anaesthesia and Intensive Care*, 2nd Edn. Oxford University Press, 1997

A 68. **A.** true **B.** false **C.** true **D.** true **E.** true

Ephedrine, a sympathomimetic amine, acts both directly (alpha- and beta-agonist) and indirectly by increasing noradrenaline release from sympathetic nerve terminals. It is a positive inotrope and chronotrope and causes an increase in systemic vascular resistance. As a beta-2 agonist, it will lead to bronchodilation. It causes uterine, bladder and GI smooth muscle relaxation. With prolonged use it displays tachyphylaxis.

Sasada M, Smith S. *Drugs in Anaesthesia and Intensive Care*, 2nd Edn. Oxford University Press, 1997

A 69. **A.** false **B.** true **C.** true **D.** false **E.** true

The volatile agents reduce uterine tone as do beta-2 agonists. Antidiuretic hormone is an octapeptide similar to oxytocin and causes uterine contraction. Prostaglandin F2-alpha is generated in large amounts by the endometrium and myometrium and acts on contractile prostaglandin F(FP) receptors to cause uterine contraction. Amyl nitrite is an organic nitrate used historically in the treatment of angina and, like other nitrates, will cause uterine relaxation.

Rang HP, Dale MM, Ritter JM. *Pharmacology*, 4th Edn. Churchill Livingstone, 1999

A. false **B.** false **C.** true **D.** false **E.** false

The sulphonylureas act mainly by augmenting insulin secretion and consequently are effective only when some residual pancreatic beta-cell activity is present. They can lead to hypoglycaemia but, unlike the biguanides, are not implicated in the production of excess lactic acid.

Pinnock CA, Lin ES, Smith T. *Fundamentals of Anaesthesia*, 2nd Edn. Greenwich Medical Media Ltd, 2003, Section 3: Chapter 14

A. true **B.** true **C.** true **D.** true **E.** false

Dextrans are polysaccharides derived from sucrose by the action of the bacterium *Leuconostoc mesenteroides* and are classified according to their average molecular weight. They are used for plasma volume replacement and in the prophylaxis of perioperative thromboembolism. They inhibit platelet adhesiveness, dilute clotting factors and dextran 40 forms a complex with fibrinogen, thereby inducing a coagulopathy. Severe hypersensitivity reactions do occur and acute renal failure has complicated the use of dextran 40 in the setting of profound hypovolaemia. They can be presented in 5% dextrose or 0.9% saline.

Hinds CJ, Watson D. *Intensive Care – A Concise Textbook*. WB Saunders, 1995

Sasada M, Smith S. *Drugs in Anaesthesia and Intensive Care*, 2nd Edn. Oxford University Press, 1997

A. false **B.** true **C.** true **D.** true **E.** false

Droperidol, a butyrophenone derivative, is used both as a neuroleptic and antiemetic. It acts as a dopaminergic (D2) receptor antagonist at the chemoreceptor trigger zone and also as a postsynaptic GABA antagonist. It has some alpha-1 antagonist properties and can cause hypotension particularly in hypovolaemic states. Extrapyramidal side effects do occur (1%) and it can cause hyperprolactinaemia. It has now been withdrawn.

Sasada M, Smith S. *Drugs in Anaesthesia and Intensive Care*, 2nd Edn. Oxford University Press, 1997

A **73.** **A.** false **B.** true **C.** false **D.** true **E.** true

Cimetidine is a reversible competitive antagonist at H2 receptors. It also has some antiandrogenic effects which may cause gynaecomastia and impotence. It is used to inhibit gastric acid secretion but has no consistent effect on lower oesophageal tone. It can reduce hepatic blood flow. An important note is that it binds to and inhibits the cytochrome P450 system and drugs metabolised by this system must be used with caution. The H1-receptor antagonists are useful in treating anaphylaxis.

Pinnock CA, Lin ES, Smith T. *Fundamentals of Anaesthesia*, 2nd Edn. Greenwich Medical Media Ltd, 2003, Section 3: Chapter 15

Sasada M, Smith S. *Drugs in Anaesthesia and Intensive Care*, 2nd Edn. Oxford University Press, 1997

A **74.** **A.** false **B.** true **C.** true **D.** false **E.** false

Midazolam is more potent than diazepam but has a shorter duration of action. It is 96% protein bound, metabolised in the liver and excreted in the urine with a elimination half-life of 2–4 h. It causes anterograde amnesia. Cerebral oxygen consumption and blood flow are reduced but their relationship maintained.

Pinnock CA, Lin ES, Smith T. *Fundamentals of Anaesthesia*, 2nd Edn. Greenwich Medical Media Ltd, 2003, Section 3: Chapter 6

Sasada M, Smith S. *Drugs in Anaesthesia and Intensive Care*, 2nd Edn. Oxford University Press, 1997

A **75.** **A.** true **B.** true **C.** false **D.** true **E.** false

Bioavailability is the amount of drug administered by a given route that reaches the systemic circulation. It is generally used in the context of orally administered drugs. Oral bioavailability of a drug will be influenced by gastric pH, enzyme activity in the GIT wall, intestinal motility and first-pass metabolism.

Pinnock CA, Lin ES, Smith T. *Fundamentals of Anaesthesia*, 2nd Edn. Greenwich Medical Media Ltd, 2003, Section 3: Chapter 2

A 76. A. true **B.** true **C.** true **D.** true **E.** true

Hyponatraemia is unusual but is a documented side effect. The thiazides act on the distal convoluted tubule to inhibit active reabsorption of sodium and chloride. There is a compensatory loss of potassium and hydrogen ions and a hypokalaemic alkalosis may develop. Calcium and uric acid secretion is reduced and blood glucose levels may rise by an enhancement of glycogenolysis and reduction in insulin secretion. Serum triglycerides and cholesterol can increase.

Rang HP, Dale MM, Ritter JM. *Pharmacology*, 4th Edn. Churchill Livingstone, 1999

A 77. A. true **B.** true **C.** false **D.** true **E.** false

Ketamine and halothane increase both cerebral blood flow and intracranial pressure.

Pinnock CA, Lin ES, Smith T. *Fundamentals of Anaesthesia*, 2nd Edn. Greenwich Medical Media Ltd, 2003, Section 3: Chapter 5

A 78. A. false **B.** true **C.** true **D.** true **E.** false

The main side effects of the aminoglycosides are ototoxicity and nephrotoxicity although nausea and vomiting, colitis, rashes, hypomagnesaemia and myasthenic syndrome have all been reported.

Pinnock CA, Lin ES, Smith T. *Fundamentals of Anaesthesia*, 2nd Edn. Greenwich Medical Media Ltd, 2003, Section 3: Chapter 18

A 79. A. true **B.** true **C.** true **D.** true **E.** false

Ketamine is effective if given by the oral, intramuscular, intravenous, extradural or intrathecal route. It stimulates respiration, is a bronchodilator and tends to preserve airway reflexes. Salivation is increased and postoperative nausea and vomiting are common. Ketamine is a racemic mixture and S(+) ketamine provides more potent analgesia than R(−) ketamine.

Pinnock CA, Lin ES, Smith T. *Fundamentals of Anaesthesia*, 2nd Edn. Greenwich Medical Media Ltd, 2003, Section 3: Chapter 6

A **80.** **A.** true **B.** true **C.** true **D.** true **E.** true

Like other volatiles, halothane will potentiate the action of non-depolarising muscle relaxants. Cutaneous vasodilation can lead to hypothermia if left unchecked. Renal blood flow is reduced by 40% and GFR by 50%. 20% of halothane is metabolised in the liver by oxidation and dehalogenation to yield trifluorocetic acid, trifluorocetylethanolamide, chlorobromodifluoroethylene and chloride and bromide radicals.

Pinnock CA, Lin ES, Smith T. *Fundamentals of Anaesthesia*, 2nd Edn. Greenwich Medical Media Ltd, 2003, Section 3: Chapter 5

Sasada M, Smith S. *Drugs in Anaesthesia and Intensive Care*, 2nd Edn. Oxford University Press, 1997

A **81.** **A.** false **B.** false **C.** true **D.** true **E.** true

Midazolam is the water soluble benzodiazepine as it has an imidazole ring in its structure which allows a conformational change with different pH conditions. The oral bioavailability of diazepam is 86–100%. Diazepam is metabolised in the liver to desmethyldiazepam (main metabolite), oxazepam and temazepam.

Sasada M, Smith S. *Drugs in Anaesthesia and Intensive Care*, 2nd Edn. Oxford University Press, 1997

A **82.** **A.** true **B.** false **C.** false **D.** false **E.** true

Mexilitine and lidocaine are used in the treatment of ventricular arrhythmias.

Pinnock CA, Lin ES, Smith T. *Fundamentals of Anaesthesia*, 2nd Edn. Greenwich Medical Media Ltd, 2003, Section 3: Chapter 12

A **83.** **A.** false **B.** false **C.** false **D.** true **E.** true

Many drugs display a Gaussian distribution of pharmacokinetic characteristics within a population. However some drug-metabolising enzymes are subject to specific genetic polymorphism. Acetylation of drugs in the liver (e.g. isoniazid) within a population shows a bimodal distribution of plasma drug concentration following a fixed dose of that drug (fast acetylators and slow acetylators). The activity of plasma cholinesterase is affected by genetic variation which can lead to an increase in the duration of action of suxamethonium.

Rang HP, Dale MM, Ritter JM. *Pharmacology*, 4th Edn. Churchill Livingstone, 1999

A 84. **A.** true **B.** true **C.** true **D.** true **E.** true

Single or repeated doses of suxamethonium can cause bradycardia. Histamine release is not uncommon and both salivation and gastric secretions are increased. Intracranial and intraocular pressures are increased. Muscle pains are particularly common in young, muscular patients.

Pinnock CA, Lin ES, Smith T. *Fundamentals of Anaesthesia*, 2nd Edn. Greenwich Medical Media Ltd, 2003, Section 3: Chapter 8

A 85. **A.** true **B.** true **C.** false **D.** false **E.** true

Atracurium is degraded both by Hoffmann elimination and some degree of ester hydrolysis. Hoffmann degradation produces laudanosine which does not have neuromuscular blocking properties but can lead to seizures. The action of non-depolarising relaxants is prolonged by hypokalaemia, hypocalcaemia, hypermagnesaemia, hypoproteinaemia, dehydration, acidosis, hypercapnia and certain drugs including alpha- and beta-blockers.

Pinnock CA, Lin ES, Smith T. *Fundamentals of Anaesthesia*, 2nd Edn. Greenwich Medical Media Ltd, 2003, Section 3: Chapter 8

A 86. **A.** true **B.** true **C.** true **D.** false **E.** true

Nitrous oxide is manufactured by heating ammonium nitrate to 240°C. Toxic impurities include nitric oxide and nitrogen dioxide. It is stored as a liquid under pressure in cylinders and the pressure is maintained until all the liquid nitrous oxide has been used. It causes cerebral vasodilation with increased cerebral blood flow and raised intracranial pressure.

Pinnock CA, Lin ES, Smith T. *Fundamentals of Anaesthesia*, 2nd Edn. Greenwich Medical Media Ltd, 2003, Section 3: Chapter 5

A 87. A. true **B.** false **C.** false **D.** true **E.** true

Bupivacaine is an amide local anaesthetic and as such is metabolised in the liver (unlike the esters which are metabolised by plasma cholinesterase). Prilocaine can lead to methaemoglobinaemia.

Pinnock CA, Lin ES, Smith T. *Fundamentals of Anaesthesia*, 2nd Edn. Greenwich Medical Media Ltd, 2003, Section 3: Chapter 9

A 88. A. true **B.** false **C.** false **D.** false **E.** false

As well as blocking sodium channels, cocaine produces blockade of the uptake-1 pathway of noradrenaline and dopamine leading to vasoconstriction.

Sasada M, Smith S. *Drugs in Anaesthesia and Intensive Care*, 2nd Edn. Oxford University Press, 1997

A 89. A. false **B.** true **C.** true **D.** true **E.** true

Halothane (2-bromo-2-chloro-1,1,1-trifluoroethane) is a halogenated ethane with a boiling point of 50.2°C. Vagal tone is increased, the automaticity of the SA node is depressed and AV conduction is delayed. Around 20% is metabolised and bromide ions may be detected in the body for weeks after prolonged exposure to halothane.

Pinnock CA, Lin ES, Smith T. *Fundamentals of Anaesthesia*, 2nd Edn. Greenwich Medical Media Ltd, 2003, Section 3: Chapter 5

A 90. A. true **B.** true **C.** false **D.** true **E.** true

Isoflurane is a halogenated methyl ether. It reduces tidal volume with little effect on respiratory rate. It has a MAC value of 1.15 (halothane 0.76) and 0.2% is metabolised (halothane 20%).

Pinnock CA, Lin ES, Smith T. *Fundamentals of Anaesthesia*, 2nd Edn. Greenwich Medical Media Ltd, 2003, Section 3: Chapter 5

A 91. A. false **B.** false **C.** false **D.** false **E.** true

Thiopentone is a thiobarbiturate presented as a yellow powder and reconstituted in water to yield a 2.5% solution with a pH of

10.8 and pKa of 7.6. It is a negative inotrope and decreases systemic vascular resistance leading to hypotension. Cerebral blood flow, intracranial pressure and intraocular pressure all fall.

Sasada M, Smith S. *Drugs in Anaesthesia and Intensive Care*, 2nd Edn. Oxford University Press, 1997

A 92. **A.** true   **B.** false   **C.** true   **D.** true   **E.** false

Nitrous oxide is a vapour with a critical temperature of 36.5°C, critical pressure of 7,260 kPa, boiling point of −88°C and blood:gas solubility coefficient of 0.47 at 37°C. Prolonged use can lead to megaloblastic anaemia, marrow aplasia and agranulocytosis.

Craft TM, Upton PM. *Key Topics in Anaesthesia*, 2nd Edn. BIOS Scientific Publishers, 1995

A 93. **A.** true   **B.** true   **C.** false   **D.** true   **E.** true

Atropine and hyoscine both cross the blood-brain barrier while glycopyrrolate does not. It increases physiological dead space and causes bronchodilation. Inhibition of sweating can lead to hyperpyrexia, particularly in children.

Sasada M, Smith S. *Drugs in Anaesthesia and Intensive Care*, 2nd Edn. Oxford University Press, 1997

A 94. **A.** false   **B.** true   **C.** true   **D.** true   **E.** true

Enflurane and isoflurane are structural isomers. Thiopentone and methohexitone display tautomerism or dynamic isomerism whereby the relative proportions of their two possible forms is determined by the surrounding pH.

Pinnock CA, Lin ES, Smith T. *Fundamentals of Anaesthesia*, 2nd Edn. Greenwich Medical Media Ltd, 2003, Section 3: Chapter 1

A 95. **A.** false   **B.** true   **C.** true   **D.** true   **E.** false

Insulin inhibits gluconeogenesis and increases the rate of glycogen synthesis by enhancing the activity of phosphofructokinase and glycogen synthetase. It causes active transport of amino acids into cells and inhibits protein catabolism. It increases the rate of potassium and magnesium transport into cells.

Sasada M, Smith S. *Drugs in Anaesthesia and Intensive Care*, 2nd Edn. Oxford University Press, 1997

A **96.** **A.** true **B.** true **C.** false **D.** true **E.** true

Etomidate, an imidazole derivative, is presented as a clear solution containing 2 mg/ml etomidate in 35% propylene glycol and water. It has a high incidence of pain on injection and has antiadrenal effects, inhibiting steroid synthesis. It lowers cerebral blood flow, intracranial pressure and intraocular pressure. It is metabolised by plasma and liver esterases and the inactive metabolites excreted in the urine.

Pinnock CA, Lin ES, Smith T. *Fundamentals of Anaesthesia*, 2nd Edn. Greenwich Medical Media Ltd, 2003, Section 3: Chapter 6

A **97.** **A.** true **B.** true **C.** false **D.** false **E.** true

	Enflurane	*Halothane*
Boiling point (°C)	56.5	50.2
SVP (kPa)	23.3	32
MAC	1.68	0.75
Molecular weight	84.5	197.4
Blood/gas solubility coefficient	1.91	2.5

Pinnock CA, Lin ES, Smith T. *Fundamentals of Anaesthesia*, 2nd Edn. Greenwich Medical Media Ltd, 2003, Section 3: Chapter 5

A **98.** **A.** true **B.** true **C.** true **D.** false **E.** true

Alfentanil, in common with other μ-agonists, is antagonised by naloxone. Compared to fentanyl its short duration of action is due to its shorter elimination half-life and smaller volume of distribution. The main metabolic pathway is N-dealkylation in the liver to form noralfentanil.

Sasada M, Smith S. *Drugs in Anaesthesia and Intensive Care*, 2nd Edn. Oxford University Press, 1997

Pharmacology

Answers

A 99. **A.** false **B.** false **C.** false **D.** false **E.** true

In the UK, oxygen is stored in black cylinders with white shoulders as a compressed gas at a pressure of 137 bar (13,700 kPa). It has a critical temperature of −118 °C, critical pressure of 50.8 atm and supports combustion but is not flammable.

Craft TM, Upton PM. *Key Topics in Anaesthesia*, 2nd Edn. BIOS Scientific Publishers, 1995

A 100. **A.** false **B.** false **C.** false **D.** false **E.** true

Carbon dioxide is stored in liquid/vapour form in grey cylinders at a pressure of 4,400 kPa. It does not support combustion (used in fire extinguishers).

Pinnock CA, Lin ES, Smith T. *Fundamentals of Anaesthesia*, 2nd Edn. Greenwich Medical Media Ltd, 2003, Section 3: Chapter 5

A 101. **A.** true **B.** false **C.** true **D.** false **E.** true

Chlorpromazine, a phenothiazine-based drug, is used as an antipsychotic, antiemetic, sedative and in the treatment of intractable hiccups. Its main therapeutic effects result from the antagonism of central dopaminergic (D2) receptors but it also has alpha blocking properties. It impairs temperature regulation.

Sasada M, Smith S. *Drugs in Anaesthesia and Intensive Care*, 2nd Edn. Oxford University Press, 1997

A 102. **A.** true **B.** false **C.** true **D.** true **E.** true

Alfentanil is the shorter acting opioid due to its smaller volume of distribution and shorter elimination half-life. The clearance of fentanyl is 13 ml/kg/min while that of alfentanil is 6 ml/kg/min. The pKa of fentanyl is 8.4, that of alfentanil 6.5. While alfentanil has a much lower lipid solubility than fentanyl it is 90% unionised in the plasma (fentanyl 9%) and therefore has a more rapid onset of action.

Calvey TN, Williams NE. *Principles and Practice of Pharmacology for Anaesthesia*, 4th Edn. Blackwell Science, 2001

A **103.** **A.** true **B.** false **C.** false **D.** false **E.** false

The oil:gas solubility coefficient determines the potency of an agent as demonstrated by the correlation between MAC values and lipid solubility. The speed of onset of an agent relates to its blood:gas solubility coefficient, a lower coefficient resulting in faster induction.

Rang HP, Dale MM, Ritter JM. *Pharmacology*, 4th Edn. Churchill Livingstone, 1999

A **104.** **A.** true **B.** true **C.** false **D.** false **E.** true

Flumazenil is a competitive antagonist at benzodiazepine receptors. Although it has some intrinsic anticonvulsant properties it has caused convulsions in epileptic patients. Dysrhythmias have been reported.

Sasada M, Smith S. *Drugs in Anaesthesia and Intensive Care*, 2nd Edn. Oxford University Press, 1997

A **105.** **A.** false **B.** false **C.** true **D.** true **E.** true

The boiling point of isoflurane is 48.5°C and MAC value is 1.15.

Pinnock CA, Lin ES, Smith T. *Fundamentals of Anaesthesia*, 2nd Edn. Greenwich Medical Media Ltd, 2003, Section 3: Chapter 5

A **106.** **A.** false **B.** false **C.** false **D.** true **E.** false

The polygelatin solutions (e.g. Haemaccel, Gelofusine) have an average molecular weight of 35,000. They do not interfere with cross-matching. In Haemaccel, the gelatin is cross-linked with urea which, when released, may be a potential problem in patients with renal failure. The half-life in the circulation of the gelatins is 4–5 h, shorter than some of the dextrans.

Hinds CJ, Watson D. *Intensive Care – A Concise Textbook*. WB Saunders, 1995

Pinnock CA, Lin ES, Smith T. *Fundamentals of Anaesthesia*, 2nd Edn. Greenwich Medical Media Ltd, 2003, Section 3: Chapter 16

A **107.** **A.** false **B.** true **C.** false **D.** false **E.** true

Oxytocin is a polypeptide secreted from the posterior pituitary. It has widespread effects including vasodilation, antidiuresis (potentially water intoxication) and milk ejection as well as uterine contraction. It is inactivated by chymotrypsin if administered orally.

Sasada M, Smith S. *Drugs in Anaesthesia and Intensive Care*, 2nd Edn. Oxford University Press, 1997

A 108. **A.** false   **B.** false   **C.** true   **D.** true   **E.** true

Heparin is a mixture of negatively-charged, acidic mucopolysaccharides. Endogenous heparin is present in the lungs, in arterial walls and in mast cells. The elimination half-life is 0.5–2.5 h.

Pinnock CA, Lin ES, Smith T. *Fundamentals of Anaesthesia*, 2nd Edn. Greenwich Medical Media Ltd, 2003, Section 3: Chapter 17

Sasada M, Smith S. *Drugs in Anaesthesia and Intensive Care*, 2nd Edn. Oxford University Press, 1997

A 109. **A.** false   **B.** true   **C.** false   **D.** true   **E.** false

Dantrolene acts within skeletal muscle to inhibit calcium release from the sarcoplasmic reticulum. It also has central GABA effects which can result in sedation. Hepatic dysfunction occurs in up to 2% of patients. Oral dantrolene is used in the prophylaxis of malignant hyperpyrexia and for the treatment of various spastic conditions.

Sasada M, Smith S. *Drugs in Anaesthesia and Intensive Care*, 2nd Edn. Oxford University Press, 1997

A 110. **A.** false   **B.** true   **C.** false   **D.** true   **E.** true

Methohexitone is a methylated oxybarbiturate which has four stereo-isomers, two of which are (or were) used commercially. When dissolved in water for injection it has a pH of 11 and pKa of 7.9. It has a high incidence of pain on injection. It is metabolised in the liver and renally excreted (<1% unchanged). It has now been withdrawn.

Pinnock CA, Lin ES, Smith T. *Fundamentals of Anaesthesia*, 2nd Edn. Greenwich Medical Media Ltd, 2003, Section 3: Chapter 6

Dantrolene is available as oral capsules and as an orange powder mixed with mannitol. It is used in the prophylaxis and treatment of malignant hyperthermia and also for the treatment of spasticity associated with chronic neurological disorders. It does not usually affect cardiac muscle or vascular smooth muscle as, in these tissues, muscle contractility is not primarily dependent on calcium release from the sarcoplasmic reticulum.

Calvey TN, Williams NE. *Principles and Practice of Pharmacology for Anaesthesia*, 4th Edn. Blackwell Science, 2001

A 112. **A.** false   **B.** true   **C.** false   **D.** true   **E.** true

Atropine is a non-selective, competitive muscarinic antagonist. It does cross the blood-brain barrier and has antiemetic properties. Like other antimuscarinics, atropine causes relaxation of visceral smooth muscle, e.g. gut, bronchi, bladder and biliary tract. Pirenzepine is a selective M-1 receptor antagonist used in peptic ulcer disease.

Rang HP, Dale MM, Ritter JM. *Pharmacology*, 4th Edn. Churchill Livingstone, 1999

A 113. **A.** false   **B.** true   **C.** false   **D.** true   **E.** true

Metoclopramide is used in the treatment of nausea and vomiting as well as migraine.

Pinnock CA, Lin ES, Smith T. *Fundamentals of Anaesthesia*, 2nd Edn. Greenwich Medical Media Ltd, 2003, Section 3: Chapter 15

A 114. **A.** true   **B.** false   **C.** true   **D.** true   **E.** true

The metabolic side effects of frusemide are numerous and include hypokalaemia, hypocalcaemia, hypomagnesaemia, hyponatraemia, hypochloraemic alkalosis, hyperuricaemia and hyperglycaemia.

Pinnock CA, Lin ES, Smith T. *Fundamentals of Anaesthesia*, 2nd Edn. Greenwich Medical Media Ltd, 2003, Section 3: Chapter 12

A 115. **A.** true   **B.** true   **C.** true   **D.** false   **E.** true

Lidocaine, an amide local anaesthetic, is a weak base with a pKa of 7.9. Amide local anaesthetics are metabolised by hepatic

Pharmacology

Answers

enzymes (amidases). In high doses lidocaine reduces systemic vascular resistance and myocardial contractility.

Calvey TN, Williams NE. *Principles and Practice of Pharmacology for Anaesthesia*, 4th Edn. Blackwell Science, 2001

A **116.** **A.** true **B.** true **C.** true **D.** false **E.** false

The pKa in isolation cannot be idealised to a precise figure as many other factors will affect the pharmacokinetic profile.

Pinnock CA, Lin ES, Smith T. *Fundamentals of Anaesthesia*, 2nd Edn. Greenwich Medical Media Ltd, 2003, Section 3: Chapter 6

A **117.** **A.** true **B.** true **C.** false **D.** true **E.** true

Hartmann's solution has a pH of 6–7 and contains:
- 131 mmol/l sodium
- 111 mmol/l chloride
- 2 mmol/l calcium
- 5 mmol/l potassium and
- 29 mmol/l lactate

Pinnock CA, Lin ES, Smith T. *Fundamentals of Anaesthesia*, 2nd Edn. Greenwich Medical Media Ltd, 2003, Section 3: Chapter 16

A **118.** **A.** false **B.** true **C.** true **D.** false **E.** true

Halothane decreases salivation and gastric motility. It causes cerebral vasodilation leading to an increase in cerebral blood flow and intracranial pressure. Its MAC value is 0.75. 20% is hepatically metabolised and the metabolites are renally excreted.

Pinnock CA, Lin ES, Smith T. *Fundamentals of Anaesthesia*, 2nd Edn. Greenwich Medical Media Ltd, 2003, Section 3: Chapter 5

A **119.** **A.** true **B.** false **C.** false **D.** true **E.** true

Lithium is normally given orally and its pharmacokinetic profile means that it takes a long time to reach a steady state and it has a long elimination half-life. It inhibits the action of ADH.

Rang HP, Dale MM, Ritter JM. *Pharmacology*, 4th Edn. Churchill Livingstone, 1999

A **120. A.** false **B.** false **C.** true **D.** false **E.** true

Many staphylococci are now resistant to some penicillins as they produce penicillinases.

Pinnock CA, Lin ES, Smith T. *Fundamentals of Anaesthesia*, 2nd Edn. Greenwich Medical Media Ltd, 2003, Section 3: Chapter 18

A **121. A.** true **B.** true **C.** false **D.** false **E.** false

Vecuronium is a monoquaternary aminosteroid which is presented as a freeze-dried, lyophilised cake for reconstitution. It does not cross the blood-brain barrier or the placenta.

Pinnock CA, Lin ES, Smith T. *Fundamentals of Anaesthesia*, 2nd Edn. Greenwich Medical Media Ltd, 2003, Section 3: Chapter 8

A **122. A.** true **B.** false **C.** true **D.** false **E.** true

Warfarin, a coumarin derivative, blocks the vitamin K dependent clotting factors. It is only effective in vivo and takes 36–48 h for the anticoagulant effect to fully develop (heparin needed in acute situation). It is 99% protein-bound, mainly to albumin and may be reversed by vitamin K.

Sasada M, Smith S. *Drugs in Anaesthesia and Intensive Care*, 2nd Edn. Oxford University Press, 1997

A **123. A.** true **B.** false **C.** true **D.** true **E.** false

Spironolactone is a synthetic steroid used in the treatment of cardiac failure, hepatic cirrhosis, nephrotic syndrome, hypertension and Conn's syndrome. It is a competitive antagonist of aldosterone in the distal convoluted tubule, increasing potassium and uric acid reabsorption and reducing sodium reabsorption. It inhibits ovarian androgen secretion and interferes with the peripheral action of androgens which can cause gynaecomastia in males. Renal blood flow and GFR are unaffected.

Sasada M, Smith S. *Drugs in Anaesthesia and Intensive Care*, 2nd Edn. Oxford University Press, 1997

A **124.** **A.** false   **B.** true   **C.** false   **D.** true   **E.** true

Vecuronium does not cross the blood-brain barrier or placenta. The volatile agents and the opioids all tend to cross the placenta.

Pinnock CA, Lin ES, Smith T. *Fundamentals of Anaesthesia*, 2nd Edn. Greenwich Medical Media Ltd, 2003, Section 3

A **125.** **A.** false   **B.** true   **C.** false   **D.** false   **E.** false

Propofol is 98% protein bound. It is conjugated in the liver by glucuronidation and then renally excreted. 0.3% is excreted unchanged in the urine.

Sasada M, Smith S. *Drugs in Anaesthesia and Intensive Care*, 2nd Edn. Oxford University Press, 1997

A **126.** **A.** false   **B.** true   **C.** true   **D.** false   **E.** true

Propofol is a white aqueous emulsion of 2,3-diisopropyl phenol (which is straw coloured) containing 10% soybean oil, 1.2% purified egg phosphatide and 2.25% glycerol. During total intravenous anaesthesia, anaesthesia is maintained at blood levels of around 3–4 mcg/kg.

Pinnock CA, Lin ES, Smith T. *Fundamentals of Anaesthesia*, 2nd Edn. Greenwich Medical Media Ltd, 2003, Section 3: Chapter 6

A **127.** **A.** true   **B.** true   **C.** false   **D.** true   **E.** false

In first order kinetics the rate of drug elimination is proportional to the plasma drug concentration. When the elimination pathways become saturated zero-order kinetics apply whereby a fixed mass of drug is eliminated in unit time irrespective of the blood concentration. Alcohol is an example of zero-order elimination.

Pinnock CA, Lin ES, Smith T. *Fundamentals of Anaesthesia*, 2nd Edn. Greenwich Medical Media Ltd, 2003, Section 3: Chapter 4

A **128.** **A.** true   **B.** true   **C.** true   **D.** true   **E.** false

Non-competitive antagonists reduce both the slope and the peak of the agonist log dose-response curve and can cause some degree of rightwards shift (non-parallel). They are non-surmountable as no matter how high an agonist concentration exists, the peak response will not be reached.

Rang HP, Dale MM, Ritter JM. *Pharmacology*, 4th Edn. Churchill Livingstone, 1999

A 129. A. false   **B.** true   **C.** true   **D.** true   **E.** true

NSAIDs inhibit cyclooxygenase which converts arachidonic to endoperoxides with subsequent release of prostaglandins, prostacyclin and thromboxane. Aspirin can displace warfarin from plasma proteins. Parecoxib is a parenteral NSAID.

Sasada M, Smith S. *Drugs in Anaesthesia and Intensive Care*, 2nd Edn. Oxford University Press, 1997

A 130. A. true   **B.** false   **C.** false   **D.** true   **E.** true

Tetracycline has a wide spectrum of antimicrobial therapy and penetrates most tissues. It is contraindicated in pregnancy and in children under 12.

Pinnock CA, Lin ES, Smith T. *Fundamentals of Anaesthesia*, 2nd Edn. Greenwich Medical Media Ltd, 2003, Section 3: Chapter 18

A 131. A. false   **B.** true   **C.** true   **D.** true   **E.** false

Naloxone can reverse the dysphoria and hypotension associated with μ-agonists. It is 91% absorbed after oral administration but undergoes extensive first-pass metabolism giving a bioavailability of 2%. Pentazocine is kappa-agonist and weak μ-antagonist.

Sasada M, Smith S. *Drugs in Anaesthesia and Intensive Care*, 2nd Edn. Oxford University Press, 1997

A 132. A. true   **B.** true   **C.** true   **D.** true   **E.** false

As a bolus, 2 mg/kg is given by slow intravenous infusion over 10–30 min.

Pinnock CA, Lin ES, Smith T. *Fundamentals of Anaesthesia*, 2nd Edn. Greenwich Medical Media Ltd, 2003, Section 3: Chapter 12

A 133. A. true **B.** true **C.** true **D.** true **E.** true

The Class 1 drugs block the voltage-sensitive sodium channels and are divided into 1a, 1b (including lidocaine) and 1c.
Class 3 drugs (amiodarone, sotalol) prolong the action potential duration and the effective refractory period. Beta-blockers normally fit into group 2 but sotalol is in group 3.

Rang HP, Dale MM, Ritter JM. *Pharmacology*, 4th Edn. Churchill Livingstone, 1999

A 134. A. true **B.** true **C.** true **D.** false **E.** true

Etomidate is an imidazole derivative presented in a propylene glycol and water solution with a pH of 8.1. It has a chiral carbon atom (and 2 isomers) and an ester bond which is metabolised by liver and plasma esterases. It does cause muscle movements and is associated with generalised epileptiform EEG activity but the link between these is not established.

Pinnock CA, Lin ES, Smith T. *Fundamentals of Anaesthesia*, 2nd Edn. Greenwich Medical Media Ltd, 2003, Section 3: Chapter 6

A 135. A. false **B.** false **C.** true **D.** true **E.** false

A clinical trial must have a hypothesis to prove or disprove and should answer as many questions as is required (the less, the better).

Pinnock CA, Lin ES, Smith T. *Fundamentals of Anaesthesia*, 2nd Edn. Greenwich Medical Media Ltd, 2003, Section 3: Chapter 19

A 136. A. true **B.** true **C.** true **D.** false **E.** true

Alfentanil is metabolised in the liver by N-dealkylation to noralfentanil. It has a pKa of 6.5.

Pinnock CA, Lin ES, Smith T. *Fundamentals of Anaesthesia*, 2nd Edn. Greenwich Medical Media Ltd, 2003, Section 3: Chapter 7

A 137. A. false **B.** false **C.** false **D.** false **E.** true

The blood:gas partition coefficient of an agent is a dimensionless ratio describing the relative amounts of a substance across a membrane when at equilibrium (partial pressures equal). It determines the speed of uptake of an agent. A low coefficient indicating a fast speed of onset. Potency relates to the oil:gas solubility coefficient. The blood:gas partition coefficients for halothane is 2.3.

Pinnock CA, Lin ES, Smith T. *Fundamentals of Anaesthesia*, 2nd Edn. Greenwich Medical Media Ltd, 2003, Section 3: Chapter 5

A 138. A. true **B.** false **C.** true **D.** false **E.** true

Oil:gas partition coefficients relate to the potency of an agent. The values are:
- Nitrous oxide – 1.4
- Halothane – 224
- Enflurane – 98
- Isoflurane – 91
- Sevoflurane – 53
- Desflurane – 19

Pinnock CA, Lin ES, Smith T. *Fundamentals of Anaesthesia*, 2nd Edn. Greenwich Medical Media Ltd, 2003, Section 3: Chapter 5

A 139. A. false **B.** true **C.** true **D.** false **E.** false

The recommended maximum doses are:
- Bupivacaine ($\pm$ adrenaline) – 2 mg/kg
- Levobupivacaine ($\pm$ adrenaline) – 2 mg/kg
- Lidocaine – 3 mg/kg
- Lidocaine + adrenaline – 7 mg/kg
- Prilocaine – 6 mg/kg
- Ropivacaine – 3.5 mg/kg

Pinnock CA, Lin ES, Smith T. *Fundamentals of Anaesthesia*, 2nd Edn. Greenwich Medical Media Ltd, 2003, Section 3: Chapter 9

A 140. A. true **B.** true **C.** true **D.** false **E.** false

Nitrous oxide was prepared and described by Joseph Priestly in 1772 and later investigated further by Humphrey Davy. It has a critical temperature of 36.5°C and is non-flammable but does support combustion. It causes cerebral vasodilation

Pharmacology

Answers

and increased intracranial pressure. The Fink effect (diffusion hypoxia) is due the diffusion of the gas into alveoli after anaesthesia causing displacement of oxygen and decreased PaO_2.

Calvey TN, Williams NE. *Principles and Practice of Pharmacology for Anaesthesia*, 4th Edn. Blackwell Science, 2001

A 141. **A.** true **B.** true **C.** false **D.** false **E.** false

MAC is the concentration of an agent in 100% oxygen that will prevent a reflex response to a standard skin incision in 50% of subjects and is a form of ED50. It is reduced by extremes of age, hypothermia, hypotension, hypothyroidism, reduced catecholamines and some drugs (e.g. sedatives, opioids, lithium). It is increased in children, hyperthermia, hyperthyroidism and high circulating catecholamines.

Calvey TN, Williams NE. *Principles and Practice of Pharmacology for Anaesthesia*, 4th Edn. Blackwell Science, 2001

A 142. **A.** false **B.** false **C.** false **D.** false **E.** false

The correct MAC values are:
- Halothane – 0.75
- Enflurane – 1.68
- Isoflurane – 1.15
- Desflurane – 6.35
- Sevoflurane – 2–2.2

Pinnock CA, Lin ES, Smith T. *Fundamentals of Anaesthesia*, 2nd Edn. Greenwich Medical Media Ltd, 2003, Section 3: Chapter 5

A 143. **A.** true **B.** true **C.** true **D.** true **E.** true

95% of nifedipine is metabolised in the liver to three inactive metabolites. Enalapril is a prodrug and is hydrolysed in the liver to enalaprilat, its active form.

Ketamine undergoes N-demethylation and hydroxylation in the liver.

Diltiazem undergoes deacetylation and demethylation in the liver followed by conjugation to active metabolites.

Etomidate is metabolised by plasma and hepatic esterases.

Pinnock CA, Lin ES, Smith T. *Fundamentals of Anaesthesia*, 2nd Edn. Greenwich Medical Media Ltd, 2003, Section 3

Sasada M, Smith S. *Drugs in Anaesthesia and Intensive Care*, 2nd Edn. Oxford University Press, 1997

A 144. **A.** false   **B.** true   **C.** true   **D.** false   **E.** false

If there is extensive tissue binding, the volume of distribution may be greater than total body water. The plasma half-life is a pharmacokinetic model and may not reflect the action at the drug effector site. Thiopentone normally has first-order kinetics but in large doses this may become zero-order.

Pinnock CA, Lin ES, Smith T. *Fundamentals of Anaesthesia*, 2nd Edn. Greenwich Medical Media Ltd, 2003, Section 3: Chapter 4

A 145. **A.** false   **B.** false   **C.** true   **D.** true   **E.** true

The starches are derived from amylopectin and have an average molecular weight that is significantly higher than that of albumin (69,000). It is hydrolysed by amylase and eliminated via the kidneys. Volume expansion can be greater than the volume infused. They can interfere with platelet function and prolong the PT, APTT and bleeding times.

Hinds CJ, Watson D. *Intensive Care – A Concise Textbook*. WB Saunders, 1995

Sasada M, Smith S. *Drugs in Anaesthesia and Intensive Care*, 2nd Edn. Oxford University Press, 1997

A 146. **A.** true   **B.** false   **C.** false   **D.** false   **E.** false

Bupivacine is an amide local anaesthetic which is contraindicated for intravenous regional anaesthesia.

The hyperbaric solution contains 80 mg/ml of glucose. 0.5% solution has 5 mg/ml.

Pinnock CA, Lin ES, Smith T. *Fundamentals of Anaesthesia*, 2nd Edn. Greenwich Medical Media Ltd, 2003, Section 3: Chapter 9

A 147. **A.** true **B.** true **C.** false **D.** false **E.** false

Etomidate is soluble in water but normally contains propylene glycol to improve stability and reduce its irritant effect. There is normally a slight drop in systemic vascular resistance and cerebral blood flow. It should be avoided in porphyria.

Calvey TN, Williams NE. *Principles and Practice of Pharmacology for Anaesthesia*, 4th Edn. Blackwell Science, 2001

A 148. **A.** false **B.** true **C.** false **D.** true **E.** true

Hoffmann elimination probably accounts for <40% of the elimination of atracurium. The metabolites do have minor neuromuscular blocking properties and bradycardia has been reported in association with its use. Degradation is slowed by hypothermia and acidosis.

Pinnock CA, Lin ES, Smith T. *Fundamentals of Anaesthesia*, 2nd Edn. Greenwich Medical Media Ltd, 2003, Section 3: Chapter 8

Sasada M, Smith S. *Drugs in Anaesthesia and Intensive Care*, 2nd Edn. Oxford University Press, 1997

A 149. **A.** true **B.** true **C.** true **D.** false **E.** false

Class 1 drugs affect phase 0 of the cardiac action potential by blocking sodium channels. They are divided into:
- Class 1a – increased action potential duration (e.g. quinidine, procainamide)
- Class 1b – reduced action potential duration (e.g. lidocaine)
- Class 1c – no effect on action potential duration (e.g. flecanide)

The beta-blockers are Class 2 drugs (sotalol in Class 3 as well).

Rang HP, Dale MM, Ritter JM. *Pharmacology*, 4th Edn. Churchill Livingstone, 1999

A 150. **A.** true **B.** true **C.** true **D.** true **E.** true

The chemoreceptor trigger zone (CTZ) lies in the area postrema outside the blood-brain barrier and possesses dopaminergic (D2) and serotonergic (5HT-3) receptors. The cannabinoids are also thought to work at the CTZ.

Domperidone has both central and peripheral (increasing gastric emptying and lower oesophageal sphincter tone) effects.

Pinnock CA, Lin ES, Smith T. *Fundamentals of Anaesthesia*, 2nd Edn. Greenwich Medical Media Ltd, 2003, Section 3: Chapter 15